DATE DUE

DEC 0 8 2007		

Demco, Inc.

D1005960

Smoking

OPPOSING
VIEWPOINTS®
DIGESTS

BOOKS IN THE
OPPOSING VIEWPOINTS DIGESTS SERIES:

Abortion
The American Revolution
Animal Rights
The Bill of Rights
Biomedical Ethics
Censorship
Child Abuse
The Civil Rights Movement
The Civil War
The Cold War
The Death Penalty
Drugs and Sports
Endangered Species
The Environment
Euthanasia
The Fall of the Roman Empire
Gangs
The Great Depression
Gun Control
Hate Groups
The 1960s
Slavery
Smoking
Teen Pregnancy
Teen Violence

Smoking

JAMES D. TORR

OPPOSING
VIEWPOINTS®
DIGESTS

Greenhaven Press, Inc., San Diego, California

Library of Congress Cataloging-in-Publication Data

Torr, James D., 1974–
    Smoking / by James D. Torr.
        p.   cm. — (Opposing viewpoints digests)
    ISBN 1-7377-0697-X (hardback : alk. paper) — ISBN 0-7377-0696-1 (pbk. : alk. paper)
    1. Smoking—United States—Juvenile literature. [1. Smoking. 2. Tobacco habit. 3. Nicotine.] I. Title. II. Series.

HV5760.T67 2001
362.29'6—dc21   00-012036

Cover Photo: Spencer Grant/Liaison International
©Catherine Karnow/Corbis: 16
PhotoDisc: 33, 42, 66, 75
©Joel W. Rogers/Corbis: 48

©2001 by Greenhaven Press, Inc.
PO Box 289009, San Diego, CA 92198-9009

Printed in the U.S.A.

CONTENTS

Foreword   6

Introduction: A Brief History of Smoking in America   8

Chapter 1: How Serious Is the Problem of Smoking?

1. Smoking Is a Serious Health Hazard   19

2. The Health Risks of Smoking Are Exaggerated   26

3. Teen Smoking Is a Serious Problem   32

4. The Problem of Teen Smoking Has Been Exaggerated   38

Chapter 2: Is the Tobacco Industry Responsible
   for the Health Consequences of Smoking?

1. The Tobacco Industry Is Responsible for
   Encouraging Smoking   45

2. Individuals Are Responsible for Choosing to Smoke   51

3. Lawsuits Against Tobacco Companies Are Justified   56

4. Lawsuits Against Tobacco Companies
   Are Not Justified   63

Chapter 3: Should the Government
   Increase Efforts to Reduce Smoking?

1. The Government Should Increase
   Efforts to Reduce Smoking   71

2. The Government Should Respect Smokers' Rights   78

Study Questions   84

Appendix A: Facts About Smoking   86

Appendix B: Related Documents   88

Organizations to Contact   97

For Further Reading   102

Works Consulted   103

Index   108

About the Author   112

FOREWORD

The only way in which a human being can make some approach to knowing the whole of a subject is by hearing what can be said about it by persons of every variety of opinion and studying all modes in which it can be looked at by every character of mind. No wise man ever acquired his wisdom in any mode but this.

—John Stuart Mill

Today, young adults are inundated with a wide variety of points of view on an equally wide spectrum of subjects. Often overshadowing traditional books and newspapers as forums for these views are a host of broadcast, print, and electronic media, including television news and entertainment programs, talk shows, and commercials; radio talk shows and call-in lines; movies, home videos, and compact discs; magazines and supermarket tabloids; and the increasingly popular and influential Internet.

For teenagers, this multiplicity of sources, ideas, and opinions can be both positive and negative. On the one hand, a wealth of useful, interesting, and enlightening information is readily available virtually at their fingertips, underscoring the need for teens to recognize and consider a wide range of views besides their own. As Mark Twain put it, "It were not best that we should all think alike; it is difference of opinion that makes horse races." On the other hand, the range of opinions on a given subject is often too wide to absorb and analyze easily. Trying to keep up with, sort out, and form personal opinions from such a barrage can be daunting for anyone, let alone young people who have not yet acquired effective critical judgment skills.

Moreover, to the task of evaluating this assortment of impersonal information, many teenagers bring firsthand experience of serious and emotionally charged social and health problems, including divorce, family violence, alcoholism and drug abuse, rape, unwanted pregnancy, the spread of AIDS, and eating disorders. Teens are often forced to deal with these problems before they are capable of objective opinion based on reason and judgment. All too often, teens' response to these deep personal issues is impulsive rather than carefully considered.

Greenhaven Press's Opposing Viewpoints Digests are designed to aid in examining important current issues in a way that develops critical thinking and evaluating skills. Each book presents thought-provoking argument and stimulating debate on a single issue. By examining an issue from many different points of view, readers come to realize its complexity and acknowledge the validity of opposing opinions. This insight is especially helpful in writing reports, research papers, and persuasive essays, when students must competently address common objections and controversies related to their topic. In addition, examination of the diverse mix of opinions in each volume challenges readers to question their own strongly held opinions and assumptions. While the point of such examination is not to change readers' minds, examining views that oppose their own will certainly deepen their own knowledge of the issue and help them realize exactly why they hold the opinion they do.

The Opposing Viewpoints Digests offer a number of unique features that sharpen young readers' critical thinking and reading skills. To assure an appropriate and consistent reading level for young adults, all essays in each volume are written by a single author. Each essay heavily quotes readable primary sources that are fully cited to allow for further research and documentation. Thus, primary sources are introduced in a context to enhance comprehension.

In addition, each volume includes extensive research tools. A section containing relevant source material includes interviews, excerpts from original research, and the opinions of prominent spokespersons. Two bibliographies, one for young adults and one listing the author's sources, are also included; both are annotated to guide student research. Finally, a comprehensive index allows students to scan and locate content efficiently.

Greenhaven's Opposing Viewpoints Digests, like Greenhaven's higher level and critically acclaimed Opposing Viewpoints Series, have been developed around the concept that an awareness and appreciation for the complexity of seemingly simple issues is particularly important in a democratic society. In a democracy, the common good is often, and very appropriately, decided by open debate of widely varying views. As one of our democracy's greatest advocates, Thomas Jefferson, observed, "Difference of opinion leads to inquiry, and inquiry to truth." It is to this principle that Opposing Viewpoints Digests are dedicated.

A Brief History of Smoking in America

The history of tobacco dates at least back to 1492, when Christopher Columbus first set foot in the New World. The American Indians he and his men encountered were fond of chewing a particular type of leaf and inhaling its smoke through a Y-shaped pipe they called a "toboca" or "tobaga." Columbus initially scolded his men for joining the natives in their custom, but finally relented. He is purported to have said that "it was not within their power to refrain from indulging in the habit."[1]

The plant was soon hailed by Europeans as one of the treasures of the New World, along with coffee, chocolate, and cane sugar. In the seventeenth century, the crop was of vital economic importance to the first English settlers in North America. Professors of geography John Fraser Hart and Ennis L. Chang note that "the colonists at Jamestown, Virginia, were exporting tobacco to England six years before the Pilgrims stepped ashore at Plymouth Rock, and for nearly four centuries the golden leaf has been one of the nation's leading cash crops."[2]

The Rise of Cigarette Smoking

Prior to the twentieth century, most tobacco was consumed in pipes and cigars or as snuff (finely pulverized tobacco inhaled into the nostrils). Cigarettes did not become popular, or even widely available, until the 1880s, when innovators such as James B. Duke developed mechanized methods of producing them. Prior to this time cigarettes had to be hand-rolled; mass production greatly reduced their price. The combination of low price and milder smoke, compared with that of pipes or cigars, greatly increased the popularity of cigarette smoking. "Per capita [per person] consumption of cigarettes rose nearly a hundredfold between 1870 and 1890, from less than one [per year] to more than 35," notes *Reason* editor Jacob Sullum. "In 1900 chewing tobacco, cigars, and pipes were still more popular, but by 1910 cigarettes had become the leading tobacco product in the United States. Per capita consumption skyrocketed from 85 that year to nearly 1,000 in 1930."[3]

As the popularity of cigarette smoking rose, so did opposition to the practice. Health advocates worried, correctly, that cigarettes were more dangerous than other forms of tobacco, because, unlike cigars and pipes, cigarette smoke is typically inhaled. Religious groups denounced cigarettes. Critics referred to them as "coffin nails" and "little white slavers." Industrialist Henry Ford spoke out against cigarettes, publishing a tract with the title *The Case Against the Little White Slaver*, and inventor Thomas Edison refused to hire smokers.

Between 1893 and 1921, in response to this antismoking sentiment, fourteen states enacted laws banning the sale, and in some cases possession, of cigarettes. Upholding Tennessee's ban in 1898, the Supreme Court declared that cigarettes "are wholly noxious and deleterious to health. . . . Beyond any question, their every tendency is toward the impairment of physical health and mental vigor."[4]

Smoking's Popularity Reaches New Heights

With the passage of the Eighteenth Amendment in 1919, the United States entered the era of Prohibition, when the sale and manufacture of alcoholic beverages were virtually banned. Throughout the 1920s and into the 1930s, however, the stubborn public enjoyed both smoking and drinking in underground speakeasies. By the start of the 1930s, most states had repealed their antismoking legislation. And by the time Prohibition was lifted in 1933, opposition to smoking had died down, and theaters, railroads, and steamships had begun to provide special smoking rooms.

In 1932 Americans elected Franklin D. Roosevelt, the first president widely known to be a cigarette smoker. During the Great Depression of the 1930s, the government enacted several programs to stabilize prices on a variety of crops, including tobacco. During World War II, cigarettes were included in soldiers' C-rations, and tobacco companies sent millions of free cigarettes to troops overseas. Many of these soldiers continued to smoke regularly when they returned home, and smoking became an accepted part of popular culture. According to the American Medical Association:

> Between the World Wars, smoking rates soared and continued to rise for decades as cigarettes became part of the popular culture, linked by manufacturers, advertisers, the entertainment industry, and the media with glamour, success, and athletic performance. Its social acceptability was unquestioned by the time of the first major challenges regarding smoking's health effects.[5]

The 1964 Surgeon General's Report

Those challenges came throughout the 1950s. Physicians began noticing that rates of lung cancer had been on the rise since 1930, and the published results of several large epidemiological studies indicated that cigarette smoking might be the cause. In response, cigarette advertisements began touting lower tar and nicotine levels, the two ingredient substances believed to be most hazardous, and tobacco companies introduced filtered cigarettes, designed to reduce the tar inhaled in smoke. In 1954, the tobacco industry ran a full-page advertisement, with the heading "A Frank Statement to Smokers," acknowledging that "experiments with mice have given wide publicity to a theory that cigarette smoking is in some way linked with cancer in human beings." The statement claimed that "there is no proof that cigarette smoking is one of the causes [of cancer]" but promised that "the fact that cigarette smoking should even be suspected as a cause of a serious disease is a matter of deep concern to us."[6]

Evidence linking lung cancer to smoking continued to accumulate, leading Surgeon General Luther Terry to release the Surgeon General's Report on Smoking and Health in 1964. Anticipating a sensational reaction, officials released the report on a Saturday to minimize its effect on the stock market and ensure coverage in the Sunday newspapers. On the basis of over more than seven thousand medical articles related to smoking and health that were already available, the report concluded that cigarette smoking is a cause of cancer and other serious diseases. "Cigarette smoking is a health hazard of sufficient importance in the United States to warrant appropriate remedial action,"[7] it warned.

"The report hit the country like a bombshell," recalls Terry. "It was front page news and the lead story on every radio and television station in the United States."[8] Indeed, the release of the landmark report seems to have marked a turning point in the nation's attitude toward smoking. In 1965, according to the Centers for Disease Control and Prevention (CDC) in Atlanta, over 42 percent of adults smoked. That figure has declined almost every year since. As of 2000, approximately 24 percent of adults smoke. (Notably, however, smoking among teens has not seen a similar decline. The CDC reports that in 1975, roughly 37 percent of high school seniors smoked; in 1997 that figure was about 36 percent.)

Government Regulation of Smoking

Since 1964 the nation's turn away from smoking has been spurred by the growing body of evidence on the dangers of smoking and the government initiatives that have followed. In 1986 the surgeon general reported that secondhand smoke can cause lung cancer, and in 1988 that cigarette smoking is addictive. Congress passed a law in 1966 requiring a warning label on cigarette packaging. Originally the label read "Caution: Cigarette Smoking May Be Hazardous to Your

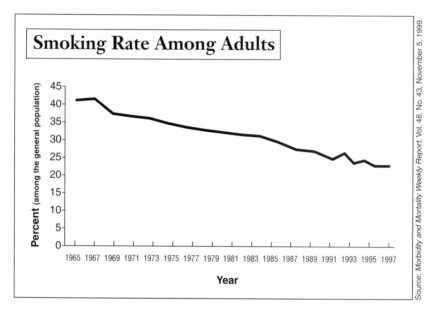

Smoking Rate Among Adults

Percent (among the general population) / Year

Health." In 1970 Congress voted to ban cigarette advertising on radio and television, a law that took effect in 1971.

State governments also passed laws to protect nonsmokers from cigarette smoke. By 1970, fourteen states had passed laws banning smoking in enclosed public places such as buses, elevators, and stores. Sometimes these restrictions came in the form of antipollution legislation. In 1975, Minnesota passed its Clean Indoor Air Act, the first comprehensive law to ban smoking in many public places, including restaurants and workplaces. Because the Minnesota law was the first to prohibit smoking *except* in specific, designated smoking areas, it is considered the first to have placed the rights of nonsmokers above those of smokers.

A series of city, state, and federal laws restricting smoking in public places has followed. The federal Department of Health, Education, and Welfare restricted smoking in federal government buildings in 1971, and as of 1999, according to the American Lung Association (ALA), only seven states do not restrict smoking in state government buildings. In 1994 the federal Pro-Children Act banned smoking in day-care centers and schools that receive federal funding. ALA also reports that thirty states have laws restricting smoking in restaurants, usually by requiring separate smoking and non-smoking areas, and three states ban smoking in restaurants entirely. In 1999, California became the first state to almost completely ban smoking in bars.

Targeting the Tobacco Industry

In addition to legislation, in the 1990s antismoking activists developed another strategy: attacking the tobacco industry directly, through the courts. Prior to 1994, tobacco companies were usually able to shield themselves from lawsuits by arguing that smokers knew the dangers of smoking and therefore, in legal terms, "assumed the risk." Ironically, their argument rested in part on the assertion that the surgeon general's warning label absolved them of legal responsibility for the diseases smoking can cause. However, in 1992 the Supreme Court ruled in *Cipollone v. Liggett Group* that some victims of smoking-related illnesses had the right to sue tobacco companies in court—for example, those who began smoking before the warning labels were in effect. Most important, the Court also ruled that tobacco companies might be held liable if it could be proved that they purposely concealed or lied about the health risks of smoking.

Evidence of exactly these charges came in 1994, when former Brown and Williamson employee Merrell Williams made public over eight thousand pages of that tobacco company's internal documents. Among other things, these documents revealed that as early as the 1960s the tobacco industry had known that nicotine was an addictive drug, that it had intentionally bred tobacco strains with higher nicotine levels, that it worked to counter evidence that smoking was dangerous, and that it opposed efforts to prevent youth smoking.

These revelations instigated a new wave of lawsuits against the tobacco companies. A novel type of lawsuit soon emerged— states began suing the tobacco industry for the medical costs of smoking-related illnesses, which are often treated under state-administered health care plans such as Medicaid. In 1994, Mississippi was the first state to sue the industry, but Minnesota's subsequent efforts proved the most groundbreaking. Minnesota state lawyers investigating the tobacco industry requested, and received, permission from Congress to gain access to thousands more of the industry's secret internal documents. These new documents provided yet more evidence of the industry's irresponsible behavior, further weakening its legal defense.

The Tobacco Wars

By mid-1997, forty states had filed lawsuits against the five major tobacco companies (Philip Morris, R.J. Reynolds, Brown and Williamson, Lorillard, and the Liggett Group). Throughout 1997, there was much talk of a possible "universal settlement" in which the industry would agree to pay the states $386.5 billion and submit to a variety of regulations concerning the marketing of cigarettes to youth, in exchange for immunity from further state lawsuits. The settlement, however, failed to gain its required congressional approval, and by September 1997 negotiations had stalled.

Instead of an out-of-court settlement, in April 1998 Arizona senator John McCain proposed federal legislation, in the form of the National Tobacco Policy and Youth Smoking Reduction Act. The McCain bill included the following provisions:

- The tobacco companies would pay $516 billion over twenty-five years into a government fund for anti-tobacco programs.
- The federal Food and Drug Administration (FDA) would be given authority to regulate tobacco products.
- Outdoor tobacco advertising, as well as cigarette ads featuring cartoon or human figures, would be banned because it has been argued that this type of advertising targets youths.

- The price of cigarettes would increase by over a dollar per pack over five years, with the revenue from increased cigarette taxes going toward smoking-prevention programs.

However, the tobacco industry objected to the stronger provisions of the McCain bill, particularly to the fact that it did not grant them immunity from further state lawsuits. The industry launched a $50 million advertising campaign against the bill, and eventually the Senate abandoned it.

Finally, in November 1998, the forty-six states that had not already settled with the tobacco companies agreed on a new settlement that was generally weaker than either of the previous proposals. The tobacco companies agreed to pay the states $209 billion over twenty-five years in exchange for immunity from further state lawsuits. The industry also agreed to ban cartoon figures, such as the controversial Joe Camel, in its advertising, and to curtail outdoor advertising and promotions aimed at youth, but some outdoor advertising would still be allowed, as would the use of human figures, such as the Marlboro Man. Worst of all, according to tobacco control activists, the FDA would not regulate tobacco.

The Current Situation

With the close of the state lawsuits against the cigarette companies, the "tobacco wars" that began in the 1990s appear to be nearing an end—although President Clinton announced in 1999 that the federal government is also planning to sue the industry to recoup the costs Medicare has incurred treating smoking-related illnesses. Many of the controversies over smoking, of course, are far from being resolved.

For example, while the evidence linking smoking to cancer has been accumulating for decades, the effects of secondhand smoke are less well understood. It is generally acknowledged that secondhand smoke contains the same carcinogens that

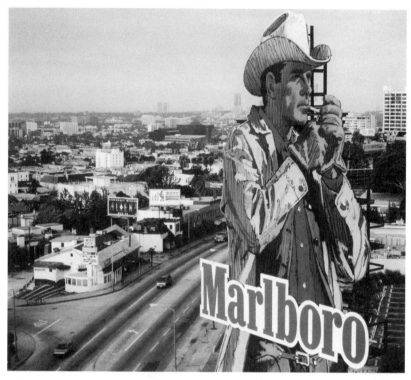

Advertisements such as this Marlboro Man billboard in Los Angeles were permitted under the November 1998 settlement, which allowed the tobacco companies to keep some outdoor advertising and the use of human figures in advertisements.

smokers inhale in so-called mainstream smoke, but it is not clear exactly how dangerous secondhand smoke is for nonsmokers. Physicians and psychologists also disagree on how addictive nicotine is.

Most of the controversies surrounding smoking, though, deal with social rather than scientific issues. How should tobacco advertising be regulated? Should tobacco be regulated as a drug? How should the problem of teen smoking be addressed? Do adults have a "right to smoke"? Does the government have the right to restrict smoking? Far more is known about the health hazards of smoking today than when smoking first became popular at the beginning of the twentieth century. But the questions of how public policy should deal with smoking have only grown more complex.

1. Quoted in *Mother Jones*, "The Tobacco Wars," May/June 1996, p. 40.

2. John Fraser Hart and Ennis L. Chang, "Turmoil in Tobaccoland," *Geographical Review*, October 1996, p. 550.

3. Jacob Sullum, "Smoke Alarm," *Reason*, May 1996, p. 40.

4. Quoted in Sullum, "Smoke Alarm," p. 40.

5. American Medical Association, *How to Help Patients Stop Smoking: Guidelines for Diagnosis and Treatment of Nicotine Dependence*. Chicago: American Medical Association, 1994, http://iumeded.med.iupui.edu/Tobacco/tobuse.htm.

6. Quoted in Stanton A. Glantz et al., *The Cigarette Papers*. Berkeley and Los Angeles: University of California Press, 1996, p. 34.

7. Quoted in Centers for Disease Control and Prevention, "History of the 1964 Surgeon General's Report on Smoking and Health," July 1996, www.cdc.gov/tobacco/31yrsgen.htm.

8. Quoted in John Parascandola, "The Surgeon General and Smoking," *Public Health Reports*, September/October 1997, p. 440.

CHAPTER 1

How Serious Is the Problem of Smoking?

"Each year . . . smoking kills more people than AIDS, alcohol, drug abuse, car crashes, murders, suicides, and fires—combined!"

Smoking Is a Serious Health Hazard

In 1964 Surgeon General Luther Terry released the first Surgeon General's Report on Smoking and Health, the first widely publicized official recognition of the dangers of smoking. On the basis of over seven thousand medical articles related to smoking and health that were already available, the report concluded that cigarette smoking is a cause of lung cancer and chronic bronchitis. "Cigarette smoking is a health hazard of sufficient importance in the United States to warrant appropriate remedial action,"[1] the report warned.

The Biggest Killer in America

In the decades since that landmark report, numerous studies have confirmed the link between smoking and lung cancer and revealed links between smoking and cancers of the larynx, oral cavity, pharynx, and esophagus, leading Surgeon General C. Everett Koop to conclude in 1982, "Cigarette smoking is the major single cause of cancer mortality in the United States."[2] The National Cancer Institute estimates that smoking alone is directly responsible for at least one-third of all cancer deaths in the United States. In addition to cancer, smoking has been shown to be a major cause of heart disease, bronchitis, emphysema, and stroke. For women, smoking is associated with poor reproductive health, including increased risk of miscarriage, preterm delivery, stillbirth, and low infant birth weight.

Smoking has such a devastating effect on the body because cigarette smoke is, in a word, toxic. There are more than four thousand chemicals in the average puff of cigarette smoke. Of these, about sixty are carcinogens—substances that can cause cancer by initiating or promoting the growth of tumors in human tissue. These chemicals include tar, carbon monoxide, ammonia formaldehyde, benzene, and nicotine. Cigarette smoke also acts as an irritant to the lungs, causing bronchial tubes to constrict and stimulating the production of mucus. This is what causes smokers to cough so much and in the long term leads to irreversible lung damage and chronic bronchitis.

Despite all that is known about the health hazards of smoking, the Centers for Disease Control and Prevention (CDC) estimates that approximately 26 percent of American adults—

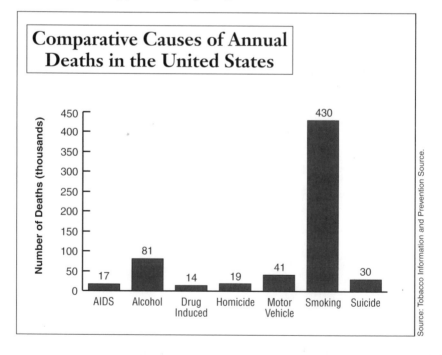

Comparative Causes of Annual Deaths in the United States

Source: Tobacco Information and Prevention Source.

some 48 million—continue to smoke, with tragic results. The CDC estimates that smoking is responsible for 430,000 (one of every five) deaths each year (compared with about 100,000 from misuse of alcohol and 20,000 from illicit drug use). "Each year," notes the CDC, "smoking kills more people than AIDS, alcohol, drug abuse, car crashes, murders, suicides, and fires—combined!"[3] Lung and other cancers account for approximately 150,000 of these deaths; heart disease, stroke, and other cardiovascular diseases account for about 180,000; and respiratory diseases such as bronchitis and emphysema account for another 85,000. "Approximately ten million people in the United States have died from smoking-attributable causes," notes the CDC. "Two million of those deaths, more than the population of Houston, have been from lung cancer alone."[4]

Nicotine Addiction

The most tragic aspect of these figures is that many of these deaths were preventable. As the American Cancer Society explains, "Smoking is the most *preventable* cause of premature death in our society."[5] Given this information, why do so many people continue to smoke? One reason is that smoking is an addictive behavior, as evidenced by the difficulty many smokers encounter in trying to quit. "It is well documented that most smokers identify tobacco as harmful and express a desire to reduce or stop using it, and nearly 35 million of them make a serious attempt to quit each year," notes the National Institute on Drug Abuse. "Unfortunately, less than 7 percent of those who try to quit on their own achieve more than 1 year of abstinence; most relapse within a few days of attempting to quit."[6]

The addictive properties of nicotine, a drug found in tobacco, account for the dependence many smokers develop. The surgeon general first concluded in 1988 that nicotine is addictive. Since that time, researchers have been working to understand the biological mechanism by which nicotine works.

When tobacco smoke is inhaled, nicotine is absorbed into the bloodstream and travels to the brain. There, scientists believe, nicotine acts on the brain much like illegal drugs such as cocaine do. Alan I. Leshner, director of the National Institute on Drug Abuse, explains: "Some of nicotine's most important effects are exerted through the very same brain circuits as those of other drugs of abuse. Researchers found nicotine, just like cocaine, heroin and marijuana, activates dopamine-containing neurons in the critical brain pathways that control reward and pleasure."[7] Eventually the smoker becomes dependent on nicotine. As psychiatry professors Jack Henningfield and Leslie M. Schuh note, this process occurs slowly, "sneaking up" on the smoker over the course of months or years:

> People do not start smoking a pack of cigarettes per day. They would likely become ill at that level of nicotine intake. Rather, they start out with low levels. Over months and years, most people progress to higher and higher nicotine intake. They become tolerant; that is, nicotine loses its effectiveness with its continued presence in the body, and it is necessary to increase the dose to maintain its effectiveness. . . . Eventually, smokers do more than simply tolerate high nicotine doses; they need continued nicotine to feel normal and function satisfactorily.[8]

"Once they have started smoking regularly," states former FDA commissioner David A. Kessler, "most smokers are in effect deprived of the choice to stop smoking."[9]

Thus, smoking is not simply a "bad habit," as many people believed for years. Nor are smokers drawn to cigarettes solely for the "pleasure" or "flavor," as the tobacco companies used to claim. Instead, nicotine is a drug that causes both psychological and physical dependence in the user. Cigarette addiction is just as real as alcoholism and other drug addictions.

Effects on Nonsmokers

Pro-tobacco groups often claim that smokers have a right to abuse their bodies with cigarettes if they choose. That might be true if the devastating effects of nicotine addiction were limited to the smoker. Unfortunately, they are not.

Nonsmokers, including children who grow up with parents who smoke, are exposed to secondhand smoke—a combination of sidestream smoke (the smoke emitted from the burning end of a cigarette, cigar, or pipe) and mainstream smoke (the smoke exhaled by the smoker). According to the National Cancer Institute, secondhand smoke "contains essentially the same compounds as those identified . . . in the smoke inhaled by the smoker."[10] The only difference is the concentration that nonsmokers are exposed to. Though secondhand smoke is less concentrated than that inhaled by smokers, research has shown it to have a significant impact on the health of nonsmokers, especially as a cause of asthma, respiratory infections, and heart disease.

In 1992 the Environmental Protection Agency (EPA) released a groundbreaking report that classified environmental tobacco smoke (ETS) as a Group A carcinogen—meaning that there is sufficient evidence to show that the substance causes cancer in humans. The EPA estimates that approximately 3,000 American nonsmokers die each year from lung cancer caused by ETS, and that 150,000 to 300,000 children under eighteen months contract pneumonia or bronchitis as a result of breathing secondhand smoke. These findings are based on the EPA's review of available medical literature and are similar to the conclusions previously drawn by the National Academy of Sciences and the U.S. surgeon general.

Other studies show the harmful effects of smoking on non-smokers. For example, Elizabeth M. Whelan, president of the American Council on Science and Health, notes that "children of smokers have higher rates of illness and more school absenteeism," and "the vast majority of childhood middle ear infections are caused by parental smoking."[11] Many government agencies besides the EPA, including the surgeon general's office, Centers for Disease Control and Prevention (CDC), National Institute for Occupational Safety and Health (NIOSH), Occupational Safety and Health Administration (OSHA), National Academy of Sciences, International Agency for Research on Cancer (IARC), and the National Toxicology Program, have concluded that secondhand smoke is a significant health hazard.

The dangers of secondhand smoke are so important because they show that smoking threatens the health of smokers and nonsmokers alike. As the EPA states, "Having a choice to take a risk for themselves should not permit smokers to impose a risk on others."[12]

Undeniable Harm

"Smokers' rights" advocates often quibble over the exact numbers of smoking-related deaths, or point out that smoking is only one of many risk factors for diseases such as lung cancer. But they cannot deny that smoking is a dangerous habit that imposes staggering costs on society in terms of chronic disease and premature deaths. The irrefutable truth is that smoking kills.

1. Quoted in Centers for Disease Control and Prevention, "History of the 1964 Surgeon General's Report on Smoking and Health," July 1996, www.cdc.gov/tobacco/31yrsgen.htm.

2. Quoted in American Cancer Society, "Cigarette Smoking and Cancer," March 30, 2000, www.cancer.org/tobacco.cigarette_smoking.html.

3. Centers for Disease Control and Prevention, "Tobacco Information and Prevention Source: Overview," www.cdc.gov/tobacco/issue.htm.

4. Centers for Disease Control and Prevention, "In the 30 Years Since the First Surgeon General's Report . . ." www.cdc.gov/tobacco/30yrs2t.htm.

5. American Cancer Society, "Cigarette Smoking and Cancer," March 30, 2000, www.cancer.org/tobacco.cigarette_smoking.html.

6. National Institute on Drug Abuse, "Nicotine Addiction," July 24, 1998, www.nida.nih.gov/researchreports/nicotine/nicotine.html.

7. Quoted in Mary E. Williams, ed., *Smoking: At Issue*. San Diego: Greenhaven Press, 2000, p. 24.

8. Quoted in Mary E. Williams and Tamara L. Roleff, eds., *Tobacco and Smoking: Opposing Viewpoints*. San Diego: Greenhaven Press, 1998, p. 34.

9. Quoted in Jacob Sullum, "Blowing Smoke About Addiction, Ability to Quit," *Reason*, May 25, 1997, www.reason.com/opeds/jacob052597.html.

10. National Cancer Institute, "Environmental Tobacco Smoke," February 14, 2000, http://cancernet.nci.nih.gov/cancer_types/lung_cancer.shtml.

11. Quoted in Carol Wekesser, ed., *Smoking: Current Controversies*. San Diego: Greenhaven Press, 1997, p. 47.

12. Environmental Protection Agency, "Setting the Record Straight: Secondhand Smoke Is a Preventable Health Risk," June 1994, www.epa.gov/iaq/pubs/strsfs.html.

"The anti-tobacco lobby is willing to play fast and loose with the facts in order to advance its political goals."

The Health Risks of Smoking Are Exaggerated

The U.S. surgeon general has determined that cigarette smoking is hazardous to your health. No one is denying this. But in their zeal, antismoking activists—with the support of government agencies—have seriously exaggerated the dangers of smoking. Anti-tobacco crusaders have overstated the health risks that smokers face, misleadingly classifying nicotine as an addictive drug on par with cocaine and heroin and grossly distorting the data concerning the effect of secondhand smoke on nonsmokers.

Deceptive Statistics

As British statesman Benjamin Disraeli quipped, "There are three kinds of lies: lies, damned lies, and statistics." Those seeking reliable information on the health effects of smoking should keep this piece of wisdom in mind. Anti-tobacco propaganda is filled with shocking statistics on smoking, but these numbers are rarely accompanied by an explanation of how they were derived.

For example, one of the most widely cited statistics about smoking is that it "kills" over four hundred thousand Americans each year. But what does this number really mean? According to the Centers for Disease Control and Prevention (CDC), the source of this statistic, over four hundred thousand deaths "are known to be caused by or associated with smoking in adults."[1] "Associated with" simply means "occurs together with." Thus the CDC figure incorporates many deaths that were not necessarily caused by smoking. "For example," writes scientist and health policy activist Rosalind B. Marimont, "if Joe Smith is obese, has high cholesterol, diabetes, a family history of heart attack, never exercises, smokes, and dies of a heart attack, the CDC attributes his death to smoking only."[2]

Determining exactly how many people die each year "because of smoking" is impossible, because many factors are responsible for conditions such as heart disease, cancer, and stroke. It is especially important to consider that smokers generally have a poorer diet than nonsmokers—perhaps because exaggerated statistics have convinced them that their smoking habit will kill them anyway.

Anti-tobacco campaigners persist nonetheless with the four hundred thousand statistic, saying that smoking does tend to lead to a "premature" death. But Marimont and Robert A. Levy, a senior fellow at the Cato Institute, a libertarian think tank, show why this claim is misleading:

> The truth is that smoking-related deaths, even under the generous definitions used by CDC, are associated with old age. Nearly 60 percent of the deaths occur at age 70 or above; nearly 45 percent at age 75 or above; and almost 17 percent at the grand old age of 85 or above! Nevertheless, without the slightest embarrassment, the public health community persists in characterizing those deaths as "premature." Regrettable, yes; premature, no.[3]

Marimont and Levy note that car accidents, suicide, and homicide kill almost one hundred thousand people annually.

The average age in these deaths is thirty-nine, according to CDC data, compared with seventy-two for "tobacco-related" deaths. Yet antismoking propaganda makes it seem as though smoking is the bigger threat.

Bogus Warnings About Secondhand Smoke

The CDC is not the only government agency to distort scientific research for the sake of the anti-tobacco crusade. In 1992 the Environmental Protection Agency (EPA) issued one of the most widely cited reports on the dangers of secondhand smoke (which it calls environmental tobacco smoke, or ETS). Among its claims were that ETS causes cancer in humans and that three thousand nonsmokers die from lung cancer caused by ETS. On the basis of this EPA report, many state, city, and county governments rushed to pass laws banning smoking in restaurants and the workplace. California even prohibits smoking in bars.

Many scientists were skeptical of the EPA report from the start. Even Elizabeth M. Whelan, a health policy activist who supports antismoking legislation, noted at the time that "the EPA has a dismal record in separating real health risks from bogus ones."[4] She was right to be wary: In 1998 a federal judge ruled that many of the EPA's findings were scien-

Smoking-Related Deaths Versus Non-Smoking-Related Deaths		
Cause of Death	Number of Deaths per Year	Mean Age at Death
Smoking-attributed	427,743	72
Motor vehicle accidents	40,982	39
Suicide	30,484	45
Homicide	25,488	32

Source: Centers for Disease Control and Prevention.

tifically groundless. Responding to a case brought by the tobacco industry against the EPA, Judge William J. Osteen of North Carolina ruled that the EPA had "committed to a conclusion before research had begun," "disregarded information and made findings on selective information," and "produced limited evidence, then claimed the weight of the Agency's research evidence demonstrated ETS causes Cancer."[5] Judge Osteen was simply recognizing what scientists knew all along: As statistician David Murray puts it, "The science on secondhand smoke is not terribly good."[6] In fact, there is no statistically significant evidence linking secondhand smoke to cancer in nonsmokers, and a 1998 study by the World Health Organization (WHO) found that nonsmokers breathing in a smoke-filled room are at no greater risk of developing lung cancer than they are breathing in a clear room.

Nicotine Should Not Be Considered a Deadly Drug

While their manipulation of statistics and other data is inexcusable, perhaps the most serious distortion of the anti-tobacco zealots has been to convince the public that smoking is an addiction and that nicotine is a dangerous drug.

There are several important differences between smoking and such conditions as alcoholism or hardcore drug use of substances such as cocaine or heroin. First, a smoker's "dependence" on cigarettes is mostly psychological. Though a heavy smoker may experience some minor physical discomfort after quitting the habit, this is nothing compared with the severe shakes, nausea, and other symptoms that alcoholics or heroin addicts experience during withdrawal. Second, nicotine is not an intoxicant like alcohol and other drugs. As Marimont explains, "Intoxicants destroy physical coordination, emotional restraint, and moral standards. . . . Nicotine does none of these things."[7]

Smoking is a bad habit, not an addiction. Individuals make a conscious choice to smoke or not to smoke. Contrary to popular belief, many regular smokers quit. Jacob Sullum, the editor of *Reason* magazine, notes, "There are about as many former smokers in the United States as there are smokers, and 90 percent of them quit on their own, without formal treatment (usually by stopping abruptly)."[8]

But if smoking is just a habit, as common sense indicates, why do so many doctors and government officials insist on calling it an addiction? To understand why, consider who benefits from calling smoking an addiction: Pharmaceutical companies develop and market nicotine patches and other devices to "cure" the addiction; psychiatrists and others profit by providing smoking cessation "therapies"; the tobacco industry profits from smokers who feel helplessly addicted and unable to quit; and smokers themselves benefit by the rationalization that nicotine, rather than their own lack of willpower, is to blame for their inability to quit smoking. And of course, if smoking is seen as some sort of social disease rather than a lifestyle choice, then the antismoking lobby seems all the more justified in legislating tobacco use.

Politics Versus Science

The anti-tobacco lobby is willing to play fast and loose with the facts in order to advance its political goals, making it difficult to determine what the true health risks of smoking are. Here are some facts that opponents of smoking routinely ignore:

- According to a 1991 study by the RAND Corporation, smoking "reduces the life expectancy of a twenty-year-old by about 4.3 years"[9]—not nearly as much as most people tend to assume.
- According to the World Health Organization, lung cancer occurs in less than 1 percent of the population. It is a very rare disease even among smokers.
- The 1964 Surgeon General's Report, the first to link smoking with lung cancer, also noted that smokers develop

Parkinson's disease at about half the rate that nonsmokers do. Subsequent research has confirmed this phenomenon.

This information is not intended to convince anyone that smoking is a healthy activity. Rather it is intended to help put the health risks of tobacco in the proper perspective, and let the scientific facts speak for themselves. "Science must not be corrupted to advance predetermined political ends," write Levy and Marimont. "Sadly, this is exactly what has transpired as our public officials fabricate evidence to promote their crusade against big tobacco."[10]

1. Quoted in Martha Perkse, "Does Smoking Really Cause over 400,000 Deaths per Year in the U.S.?" www.forces.org/evidence/files/martha2.html.

2. Rosalind B. Marimont, "War on Smoking," 1997. Brochure distributed by FORCES USA, www.forces.org/articles/files/roz-03.htm.

3. Robert A. Levy and Rosalind B. Marimont, "Blowing Smoke About Tobacco-Related Deaths," *Cato Today's Commentary*, April 29, 1999, www.cato.org/dailys/04-29-99.html.

4. Quoted in Carol Wekesser, ed., *Smoking: Current Controversies*. San Diego: Greenhaven Press, 1997, p. 40.

5. Quoted in Robert A. Levy and Rosalind B. Marimont, "Lies, Damned Lies, and 400,000 Smoking-Related Deaths," *Regulation*, April 1999, p. 25.

6. Quoted in Jay Nordlinger, "Secondhand Statistics," *Weekly Standard*, August 3, 1998, p. 14.

7. Marimont, "War on Smoking."

8. Jacob Sullum, "Blowing Smoke About Addiction, Ability to Quit," *Reason*, May 25, 1997, www.reason.com/opeds/jacob052597.html.

9. Quoted in Levy and Marimont, "Lies, Damned Lies, and 400,000 Smoking-Related Deaths," p. 27.

10. Levy and Marimont, "Blowing Smoke About Tobacco-Related Deaths."

"If adolescents can be kept tobacco-free, most will remain tobacco-free for the rest of their lives."

Teen Smoking Is a Serious Problem

Teen smoking is a pediatric disease of epidemic proportions. The U.S. Department of Health and Human Services estimates that more than 4 million kids age twelve to seventeen smoke cigarettes. The Centers for Disease Control and Prevention (CDC) estimates that each day more than three thousand children and teenagers become regular smokers, for a total of more than 1 million new smokers a year. Adult smoking dropped steadily from the 1960s to 1990, from about 40 percent to 26 percent, but rates of teen smoking remained steady throughout the 1980s and rose in the 1990s. In 1997, according to the University of Michigan's Monitoring the Future study, the proportion of high school seniors who smoked reached a nineteen-year high of 36.5 percent. And approximately one-third of these teen smokers will die of tobacco-related illness, according to the CDC.

Addiction to Smoking Usually Begins Before Age Twenty

"Tobacco may not kill until middle age or later," writes Anne Platt McGinn, a research associate at the Worldwatch Institute, "but in a sense, it chooses its victims young. Some 90 percent of all smokers have their first cigarette by age 20."

In fact, the CDC estimates that among U.S. adults who have ever smoked daily, 91 percent tried their first cigarette and 77 percent became daily smokers before age twenty. And the younger they start smoking, the more likely children and teens are to develop smoking-related illnesses later in life. "On average," writes McGinn, "smokers who light their first cigarette at 25 lose about 4 years of life; those who start at age 15 lose 8 years."[1]

On the other hand, notes Joseph A. Califano Jr., president of the National Center on Addiction and Substance Abuse at Columbia University, "A child who gets through age 21 without smoking . . . is virtually certain never to do so."[2] This is why combating teen smoking is so important. As a 1994 surgeon general's report on tobacco and youth concludes, "If adolescents can be kept tobacco-free, most will remain tobacco-free for the rest of their lives."[3]

The CDC estimates that every day more than three thousand children and teens become regular smokers. Further, the CDC claims that the earlier young people start smoking, the greater their chances of developing smoking-related illnesses.

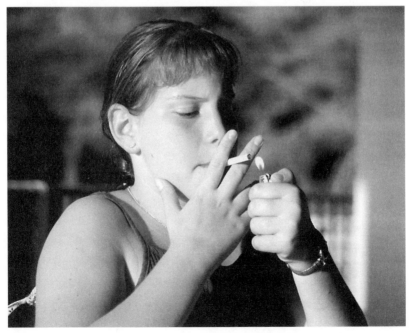

Smoking, Drinking, and Drug Use

According to a 1994 report from the surgeon general's office, "Nicotine dependency through cigarette smoking . . . is the most common form of drug addiction."[4] Cigarette smoking is not intoxicating in the way that heroin or marijuana are, but nicotine is actually stronger in terms of addiction. Young people develop a tolerance for, and become dependent on, nicotine just as quickly as adults do, and young people have just as hard a time quitting. Yet most teens do not believe that cigarettes carry the same addictive potential as illegal drugs. They may choose to smoke believing that nicotine is "safe" in comparison with other drugs, but in fact many more people die from tobacco-related illnesses than from alcohol or illegal drugs, according to the CDC.

Moreover, research indicates that smoking is associated with underage drinking and other illegal drug use as well as unhealthy and antisocial behavior. "Nicotine is generally the first drug used by young people who use alcohol, marijuana, and harder drugs,"[5] notes a 1994 surgeon general's report. A 1998 survey by the National Center on Addiction and Substance Abuse (CASA) at Columbia University found that teens who smoke are 5 1/2 times more likely to have tried marijuana, 6 times likelier to get drunk at least once a month, and 3 times likelier to try an illegal drug in the future than teens who don't smoke. CDC research also found that teens who smoke are 22 times more likely to use cocaine. Other studies have found an association between tobacco use and fighting, carrying weapons, performing poorly in school, and engaging in high-risk sexual behavior.

Why Teens Smoke

There is a variety of reasons why teens begin smoking. Advertising, along with television and movies, has glamorized smoking, making it seem like a sophisticated "adult" activity. Susan S. Lang and Beth H. Marks, authors of *Teens and*

Tobacco: A Fatal Attraction, write, "Kids are vulnerable to smoking because the transition to adulthood is fraught with stress, insecurity, and the need to be accepted by peers. If kids see smokers who they think are cool or look grown-up, they may strive for that image, too."[6] Many teens try their first cigarette to fit in with a peer group. Some teenage girls believe that smoking can help them lose or keep off weight. And of course, many teens smoke to rebel against parents, teachers, or society in general.

Tobacco companies are well aware of the various appeals that smoking has for teens—and work to exploit them and encourage teenagers to smoke. Each year Big Tobacco loses—and therefore must replace—over 2 million customers, either because they quit smoking or because they die. Although the tobacco companies repeatedly proclaim that they no longer intentionally market cigarettes to children, the fact remains: Most new smokers are teenagers.

Combating Teen Smoking

Teenagers are the largest group of nonsmokers who are most likely to begin smoking and become addicted. It follows that efforts to reduce and prevent smoking should target teens.

The first step in combating teen smoking is to reduce teens' access to tobacco. One way to reduce smoking, among both teens and adults, is to raise taxes on tobacco products: The more expensive cigarettes are, the fewer people will buy. Another easy-to-implement method of reducing minors' access to tobacco would be to ban cigarette vending machines, which give children of any age easy access to tobacco.

But many teens are able to buy cigarettes over the counter, despite the fact that all fifty states prohibit the sale of cigarettes to minors. The Campaign for Tobacco-Free Kids estimates that about half of all underage smokers buy cigarettes for themselves. If state and local governments are unwilling or unable to ensure that laws prohibiting the sale of cigarettes to minors are enforced, the federal government may have to step in. One way to give the federal government the ability to enforce these laws would be to give the Food and Drug Administration (FDA) the authority to regulate nicotine as a drug. Unfortunately, the Supreme Court ruled in March 2000 that the FDA does not have the authority to regulate tobacco. But this does not rule out the possibility that a comprehensive federal program for tobacco control could be enacted if states are unable to control minors' access to tobacco.

In addition to physically restricting minors' access to tobacco, effective smoking-prevention programs must educate children and teens about the dangers of tobacco and teach them how to resist social pressures to smoke. These programs should emphasize the dangers of smoking, both in terms of its addictive nature and the long-term health problems it causes. Antismoking campaigns should also work to deglamorize smoking, thus serving as an antidote to smoking advertisements and movies in which attractive actors smoke. Finally, in order to debunk the notion that smoking is an act of rebellion, antismoking efforts should emphasize how teen smoking profits cigarette manufacturers at the expense of unsuspecting teens. As *Boston Globe* columnist Ellen Goodman puts it, kids must be shown that "they are being manipulated, not liberated, by CEOs in suits."[7]

Public service advertisements and educational programs in many states have emphasized precisely these points. But more needs to be done: The CDC estimates that, if current trends continue, approximately 5 million children and teens who are alive today will die from tobacco-related illnesses. As Lang and Marks write, "It is kids who feed [the] epidemic of smoking."[8]

1. Anne Platt McGinn, "The Nicotine Cartel," *Worldwatch*, July/August 1997, p. 20.

2. Joseph A. Califano Jr., opening address at Substance Abuse in the 21st Century: Positioning the Nation for Progress, Simi Valley, California, March 1, 2000, www.casacolumbia.org.

3. Centers for Disease Control and Prevention, "Preventing Tobacco Use Among Young People: A Report of the Surgeon General: At-a-Glance," 1994, www.cdc.gov/tobacco/ 94oshaag.htm.

4. Quoted in Susan S. Lang and Beth H. Marks, *Teens and Tobacco: A Fatal Attraction.* New York: Twenty-First Century Books, 1996, p. 88.

5. Centers for Disease Control and Prevention, "Preventing Tobacco Use Among Young People."

6. Lang and Marks, *Teens and Tobacco*, p. 11.

7. Ellen Goodman, "Whining Tobacco Companies Still Targeting Youth," *Liberal Opinion Week*, April 20, 1998.

8. Lang and Marks, *Teens and Tobacco*, p. 11.

"Cigarettes do not kill a single young person."

The Problem of Teen Smoking Has Been Exaggerated

Smoking is bad for one's health. Health-conscious adults should not smoke (although in a free society they cannot be prohibited from doing so). Smoking is especially bad for children and adolescents, since it is bad for the lungs and can develop into a lifelong habit. It is perfectly reasonable for parents to discourage or prohibit their children from smoking. That said, the current hysteria over teen smoking is very far from reasonable. The problem of teen smoking is simply not worth the crusade society is waging against it.

The Prevalence of Teen Smoking Is Exaggerated

The vast majority of smokers—well over 90 percent—are adults who have the right to smoke if they choose. Unable to dispute this fact, antismoking activists have chosen to focus on smokers age seventeen and under. According to the Department of Health and Human Services, there are approximately 4 million underage smokers in the United States, compared with the estimated 48 million adult smokers. The University of Michigan's Monitoring the Future study found that about 34.9 percent of high school seniors were smokers in 1999 (down from 36.5 percent in 1997).

Of course, the reliability of any statistic varies with the source. Antismoking activists are certainly willing to quote numbers that have little basis in reality. For example, one popular figure is that each day three thousand children begin to smoke. This number appears prominently on the website of the Campaign for Tobacco-Free Kids and has been quoted by numerous politicians, including President Bill Clinton. But what is the source of this staggering number? According to Jay Nordlinger, associate editor of the *Weekly Standard*, "The 3,000 figure on kids began in 1989, when the *Journal of the American Medical Association* published 'Trends in Cigarette Smoking in the United States.' The authors found that '1 million new young persons per year are recruited to the ranks of regular smokers,' the equivalent of 'about 3,000 new smokers each day.'"[1]

But the authors of the study clearly state, "For purposes of this analysis, only persons aged 20 years and older are included, as information was not collected on younger persons in any consistent fashion."[2] Thus the three-thousand-a-day figure

Source: Institute for Social Research, University of Michigan, Monitoring the Future Project.

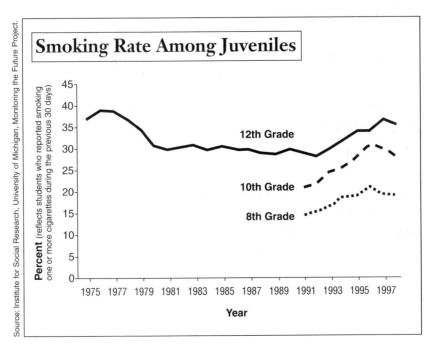

Smoking Rate Among Juveniles

refers to *twenty-year-olds*. The study, originally published in 1989, has been quoted and requoted: Along the way someone changed the term "young persons" to "children." This type of distortion is common in the antismoking literature.

Bombarding Children with Antismoking Propaganda

The exact number of teen smokers is irrelevant, reply the anti-tobacco crusaders; any level of underage smoking is evidence that more smoking-prevention efforts are needed. These efforts take the form of billboards and radio and television public service spots designed to brainwash children and teens into believing that cigarettes, smokers, and most of all the tobacco companies are evil.

These antismoking campaigns are problematic in several ways. The first is that teaching children not to smoke is a job for parents, not the government. The government has no business telling children that smoking—a legal activity that their parents might enjoy themselves—is unwise, unattractive, or immoral. Another problem with these campaigns is that they are funded with taxpayers' money. In California and several other states, they are funded with the revenue from cigarette taxes. There is no reason adult smokers should be forced to pay for such programs.

But the most objectionable aspect of these antismoking campaigns is their overzealousness. Antismoking advertisements routinely demonize tobacco companies, ridicule and disparage smokers, and exaggerate the dangers of smoking. "One particularly irresponsible aspect of the war against tobacco is the now commonplace equation of tobacco with drug use," writes Dennis Prager, a theologian and talk-show host in Los Angeles. Anti-tobacco billboards in several states emphasize that nicotine is an addictive drug, no different than marijuana, heroin, or cocaine. This ludicrous claim has a terrible effect on young people. "If taking heroin, cocaine, or marijuana is the moral, personal, and social equivalent of smoking cigarettes, then how bad can heroin, cocaine, and marijuana be?" asks Prager rhetorically. "After all, young people see adults smoking cigarettes all the time without destroying their lives."[3]

Exaggerating the Tobacco Threat

The truth is that smoking is simply not as grave a threat to young people as antismoking crusaders proclaim. Teenagers face many more serious problems than smoking, such as poverty, violence, and alcohol and illegal drug abuse. In fact it is misleading to characterize smoking as a "teen" issue. "Unlike drugs, drunk driving, and murder, which annually kill many thousands of young people, cigarettes do not kill a single young person," writes Prager. "Those people who die from cigarettes will do so at an average age of over 70."[4] As libertarian writer Robert A. Levy and health policy activist Rosalind B. Marimont explain, "The unvarnished fact is that children do not die of tobacco-related diseases. If they smoke heavily during their teens, they may die of lung cancer, fifty or sixty years from now, assuming lung cancer is still a threat by then. No matter how you slice it, a high-intensity government campaign against tobacco—in the guise of 'protecting children'—is disingenuous at best."[5]

A Misguided Strategy

The war against teen smoking is not only intellectually dishonest but may actually worsen the problem it seeks to reduce. James Taranto, an editor of the *Wall Street Journal*, explains why: "All teenagers instinctively recoil at being told what to do—a fact that seems to have escaped the notice of anti-smoking zealots. Their heavy-handed moralizing has made cigarette smoking into the ultimate act of adolescent rebellion, at once countercultural and politically incorrect."[6] The more teens are told not to smoke, the more they are attracted to it as a "forbidden fruit."

There is evidence that this is precisely what is happening. According to data from the Centers for Disease Control and

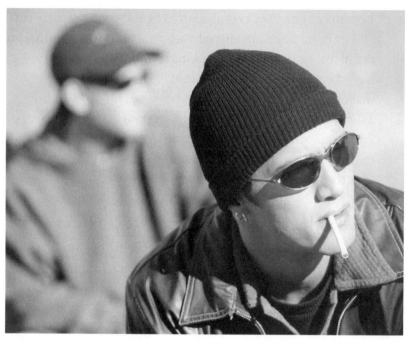

Some observers maintain that teens may choose to smoke as a way to rebel against the norm, and efforts to discourage them from smoking may in fact make cigarettes seem more appealing.

Prevention (CDC), smoking rates among adults have been declining in America since the 1960s. Teen smoking rates, however, rose significantly between 1991 and 1997—precisely the years that the modern war on tobacco was getting underway. In January 1999 the *Los Angeles Times* noted that "in a state [California] that bans smoking in restaurants and bars—and where an increasing number of cities outlaw billboards advertising cigarettes—teenage smoking rates continue to rise."[7]

Smoking among teenagers is an undesirable fact of life. But teen smoking is not a problem of epidemic proportions. Nor does smoking kill a single teenager or child. Teen smoking should be discouraged when possible, *within reasonable limits*. But antismoking activists continue to exaggerate the problem, while simultaneously claiming that new government programs can solve it. Wanda Hamilton of the National Smokers Alliance describes the situation this way:

For more than 30 years, researchers and tobacco control experts have attempted to find a solution to the problem of underage smoking. Billions of dollars have been spent. Countless studies and surveys have been conducted. Numerous programs and approaches have been tried, from school-based anti-tobacco education programs to the banning of tobacco advertising. All apparently to no avail, because today's youth smoking rates are as high as they were 20 years ago. . . .

What is the answer to stopping youth smoking? The facts show that the solution may lie in more involvement by parents, rather than more government programs and more tax dollars.

Ah, parenting. What a novel idea.[8]

1. Jay Nordlinger, "Secondhand Statistics," *Weekly Standard*, August 3, 1998, p. 15.

2. Quoted in Nordlinger, "Secondhand Statistics," p. 15.

3. Dennis Prager, "The Soul-Corrupting Anti-Tobacco Crusade," *Weekly Standard*, July 20, 1998, p. 17.

4. Prager, "The Soul-Corrupting Anti-Tobacco Crusade," p. 19.

5. Robert A. Levy and Rosalind B. Marimont, "Blowing Smoke About Tobacco-Related Deaths," *Cato Today's Commentary*, April 29, 1999. www.cato.org/dailys/04-29-99.html.

6. James Taranto, "An Adolescent View of Smoking," *American Enterprise*, September/October 1998, p. 13.

7. Quoted in Wanda Hamilton, "What Shall We Do About the Kids?: A Selected Bibliography on Underage Tobacco Use," National Smokers Alliance, 1999, www.smokersalliance.org/hamilton1.html.

8. Wanda Hamilton, "What Shall We Do About the Kids?"

CHAPTER 2

Is the Tobacco Industry Responsible for the Health Consequences of Smoking?

"Tobacco marketing . . . is what starts adolescents down the slippery slope of addiction."

The Tobacco Industry Is Responsible for Encouraging Smoking

"What makes cigarettes the most successful product in American history?" asks William Everett Bailey in his book *The Invisible Drug*. The answer: "Advertising."[1] According to the office of the surgeon general, tobacco companies spent a whopping $6.7 billion on marketing their products in 1998. "Among all U.S. manufacturers," notes Surgeon General David Satcher, "the tobacco industry is one of the most intense in marketing its products. Only the automobile industry markets its products more heavily."[2]

Tobacco Industry Denials

Big Tobacco often claims its advertisements are designed only to provide adults with "information" about smoking or to entice established smokers into switching brands. The industry would have the public believe that advertising plays no role at all in an individual's decision to smoke. But obviously the decision to smoke is influenced by many factors, and advertising is one of them. Simply put, cigarette advertising encourages people to smoke.

The fact that Big Tobacco insists that tobacco advertising only promotes brand switching among established smokers, and doesn't affect total tobacco consumption, is evidence of the deception that characterizes the industry. The fallacy of its "brand switching only" position is clearly explained by Emerson Foote, former chairman of the advertising agency McCann-Erickson:

> The cigarette industry has been artfully maintaining that cigarette advertising has nothing to do with total sales. This is complete and utter nonsense. The industry knows it is nonsense. I am always amused by the suggestion that advertising, a function that has been shown to increase consumption of virtually every other product, miraculously fails to work for tobacco products.[3]

Guy Smith, a former Philip Morris public relations executive, admits the truth: "The top three reasons people smoke are 1) Advertising, 2) Friends smoke, and 3) Family members smoke."[4]

Targeting Teens

The tobacco industry is well aware that it needs to replace the over four hundred thousand U.S. smokers who yearly either quit smoking or die, often prematurely from smoking-related illnesses. It turns to teenagers to recruit new customers. Big Tobacco knows that over 80 percent of smokers start before age eighteen, and almost no one begins smoking after age twenty. The Campaign for Tobacco-Free Kids paints an accurate picture of the tobacco business: "No matter what the cigarette companies say or do, they cannot stay in business unless kids smoke. . . . If large numbers of kids did not try smoking, become regular users, and turn into addicted adult smokers, the big cigarette companies would eventually not have enough adult customers to make staying in business worthwhile."[5]

Tobacco companies have recognized this for decades. A 1979 Philip Morris memo boasts, "Marlboro dominates in the 17 and under age category, capturing over 50% of this market." A 1973 Brown and Williamson memo recognizes that

"[The cigarette brand] Kool has shown little or no growth in share of users in the 26+ age group. Growth is from 16–25 year olds," and recommends a marketing strategy: "All magazines will be reviewed to see how efficiently they reach this group."[6] A 1978 Lorillard Tobacco document bluntly states, "The basis of our business is the high school student." As recently as 1981 a Philip Morris memo explained, "Today's teenager is tomorrow's potential regular customer, and the overwhelming majority of smokers first begin to smoke while still in their teens. . . . The smoking patterns of teenagers are particularly important to Philip Morris."[7]

These documents, made public through lawsuits against the tobacco companies in the 1990s, are dismaying proof that for decades Big Tobacco purposely—and illegally—marketed cigarettes to minors. With these immoral marketing practices, Big Tobacco helped hook millions of Americans on nicotine when they were still minors. The tragic consequences of hooking teens on smoking—lung cancer, emphysema, heart disease, etc.—do not manifest themselves until decades later, but the tobacco industry must nevertheless be held accountable for its flagrant, unscrupulous efforts to sell tobacco to children.

Big Tobacco Hasn't Changed Its Ways

Of course, Big Tobacco is also aware that peddling cigarettes to children has given it a rather villainous image, which could hurt profits. So it has promised to change its ways. Under a 1998 settlement with forty-six states that had sued the tobacco industry, the five major tobacco companies agreed to several advertising restrictions. For example, the agreement restricts advertising on billboards and bans the use of cartoon figures, such as Joe Camel, in advertising. It also prohibits brand-name sponsorship of most, but not all, concerts and sporting events.

But the settlement fell far short of a true ban on youth marketing of tobacco. For example, outdoor advertising is still permitted on buildings where tobacco is sold, even those near schools. Internet and direct-mail advertising remain completely

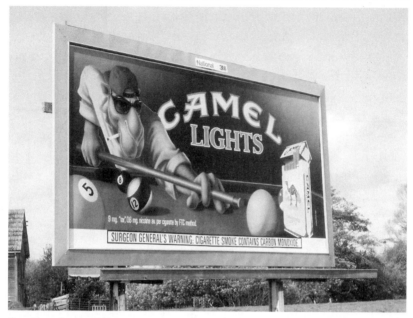

Joe Camel plays pool on an R.J. Reynolds billboard advertisement for Camel cigarettes. The use of cartoon characters, including Joe Camel, was banned as part of a 1998 legal settlement.

unrestricted. And there are no limits on cigarette ads in newspapers and magazines, even those with a large number of youth readers.

Furthermore, there is plenty of evidence that tobacco companies are continuing their youth marketing practices, despite the restrictions. While R.J. Reynolds's Joe Camel is gone, the cowboy figure of the Marlboro Man remains one of Philip Morris's most popular icons. Tobacco companies continue to favor hip, youth-oriented magazines like *Rolling Stone* for their ads. In late 1999, R.J. Reynolds debuted vanilla, citrus, and spice Camel cigarettes, flavors the industry has long believed would appeal to early smokers. Matthew Myers, director of the Campaign for Tobacco-Free Kids, said of the move, "The only way to interpret it is as yet another tobacco industry appeal to the young." "The only thing that's changed is the rhetoric," Myers says of Big Tobacco's promises. "The tobacco companies haven't changed their marketing behavior at all."[8] But again, this is not surprising, since Big Tobacco needs to hook teens to survive.

Ads Persuade Teens to Start Smoking

The sad fact is that Big Tobacco continues to aim its advertising at teens because it works. For example, a study in the *Journal of Marketing* found that Marlboro, the most heavily advertised cigarette brand, constitutes almost 60 percent of the youth market but only 35 percent of the adult market. The Centers for Disease Control and Prevention (CDC) reports that 86 percent of teen smokers prefer Marlboro, Camel, and Newport—the three most heavily advertised brands. After R.J. Reynolds introduced the Joe Camel character in 1988, Camel's share of the adolescent market increased from less than 1 percent to more than 13 percent by 1993, according to the surgeon general's office. And a study by the National Cancer Institute found that peer pressure and the example of family members who smoke are not nearly as powerful as advertising in prompting the smoking urge among teens. "Tobacco marketing . . . is what starts adolescents down the slippery slope of addiction,"[9] says Dr. John Pierce of the University of California, a coauthor of the study.

Cigarette advertisements work by trying to change people's attitudes about smoking. They create the impression that cigarettes can give people the things they want. For example, ads featuring the Marlboro Man imply that cigarettes can help make men tougher or more independent. Ads aimed at women imply that smoking can give them a sense of success, recognition, and equality with men. And ads aimed at teenagers associate smoking with a variety of things teens desire: popularity, acceptance, rebellion, sex appeal, adventure, or adulthood. Finally, ubiquitous images of people smoking convey a general sense that smoking is a normal, even healthy, activity. "Words such as *light, mild, clean, fresh, soft,* and *natural* promote this image as well,"[10] note Susan S. Lang and Beth H. Marks in their book *Teens and Tobacco: A Fatal Attraction.*

Big Tobacco Must Be Held Accountable

"We shouldn't advertise something we know to be a poison and a killer,"[11] said former surgeon general Joycelyn Elders in 1994. But marketing a cancer-causing substance to kids is exactly what the tobacco business is doing. A 2000 report from the surgeon general states, "Regulation of advertising and promotion, particularly that directed at young people, is very likely to reduce both prevalence and uptake of tobacco use."[12] However, Big Tobacco has shown a remarkable willingness to sidestep and disobey such regulations. If the tobacco industry insists on hooking teens on cigarettes with irresponsible marketing practices, they should be held liable in court.

1. Quoted in Mary E. Williams, ed., *Smoking: At Issue*. San Diego: Greenhaven Press, 2000, p. 50.

2. David Satcher, "The Surgeon General's Report on Reducing Tobacco Use: Tobacco Advertising and Promotion Fact Sheet," 2000, www.cdc.gov/tobacco/sgr_tobacco_pdf/TobaccoAdvertising.pdf.

3. Quoted in Mary E. Williams and Tamara L. Roleff, eds., *Tobacco and Smoking: Opposing Viewpoints*. San Diego: Greenhaven Press, 1998, p. 90.

4. Quoted in Williams, *Smoking*, p. 50.

5. Campaign for Tobacco-Free Kids, "The Cigarette Companies Cannot Survive Unless Kids Smoke," July 18, 2000, http://tobaccofreekids.org/research/factsheets/pdf/0012.pdf.

6. Quoted in David Tannenbaum, "Smoking Guns I: Marketing to Kids," *Multinational Monitor*, July/August 1998, p. 22.

7. Campaign for Tobacco-Free Kids, "The Cigarette Companies Cannot Survive."

8. Quoted in Marianne Lavelle, "Teen Tobacco Wars," *U.S. News & World Report*, February 7, 2000, p. 14.

9. Quoted in *Minneapolis Star-Tribune*, "Study Links Marketing, Teen Smoking," October 18, 1995, p. 4A.

10. Susan S. Lang and Beth H. Marks, *Teens and Tobacco: A Fatal Attraction*. New York: Twenty-First Century Books, 1996, p. 43.

11. Quoted in *Minneapolis Star-Tribune*, "Study Links Marketing, Teen Smoking," p. 4A.

12. David Satcher, "The Surgeon General's Report on Reducing Tobacco Use."

"People know—and have known for decades—that smoking is risky, but many of them choose to do it anyway."

Individuals Are Responsible for Choosing to Smoke

In 1994, U.S. tobacco companies were being sued by five states—Florida, Massachusetts, Minnesota, Mississippi, and West Virginia—in part on the grounds that tobacco companies were responsible for the health-care costs of lung cancer and other tobacco-related diseases. By 1997, the number of state plaintiffs had reached twenty-five, with more states joining in each month. Then in November 1998, forty-six states agreed to a massive out-of-court settlement with the five major tobacco companies—Philip Morris, R.J. Reynolds, Brown and Williamson, Lorillard, and the Liggett Group. The tobacco companies agreed to pay the states $206 billion, and to restrict their advertising practices, in exchange for immunity from further lawsuits from the states.

The multistate tobacco settlement, however, did not grant the tobacco industry immunity from private lawsuits. In February 1999, a California jury ordered Philip Morris to pay a staggering $51.5 million to Patricia Henley, who contracted lung cancer after smoking three packs of cigarettes a day for thirty-six years. On July 14, 2000, in a class-action lawsuit, a Florida judge ordered the five major tobacco companies to pay $145 billion to over seven hundred thousand smokers on the grounds that the industry had misled the public about the health risks of smoking. The decision is being appealed.

At the heart of these lawsuits is the idea that tobacco companies—and not individuals—are responsible for the health consequences of smoking. But the decision to smoke is an individual choice, and individuals must be held responsible for it.

Blaming the Tobacco Companies

Defenders of the tobacco lawsuits say the tobacco industry covered up knowledge of the harmful effects of tobacco. In essence they are saying that smokers were unaware of the dangers of smoking. Patricia Henley's lawyers, for example, argued that she took up the habit before cigarette packages carried warning labels. But warnings of the dangers of cigarettes date back to the nineteenth century; as early as 1865, manuals of the American Law Institute stated that the hazards of tobacco were common knowledge. "Until 1997," writes Jacob Sullum, senior editor of *Reason* magazine, "California blocked smokers from suing tobacco companies for the same reason."[1] California lifted that ban because of political pressure from antismoking activists. Nevertheless, the idea that any smoker could be ignorant of the fact that smoking is an unhealthy activity is preposterous. The indisputable truth is that people know—and have known for decades—that smoking is risky, but many of them choose to do it anyway.

Blaming Advertising

Another claim that anti-tobacco lawyers have made is that smokers have been "lured into" smoking by advertising. Thus not only were smokers completely ignorant of the dangers of smoking, they only took up the habit because billboards and other print advertisements told them to. This argument is usually advanced by adults who began smoking as teenagers. Anti-tobacco activists readily accept the idea that all teen smokers have been duped by advertisements featuring the car-

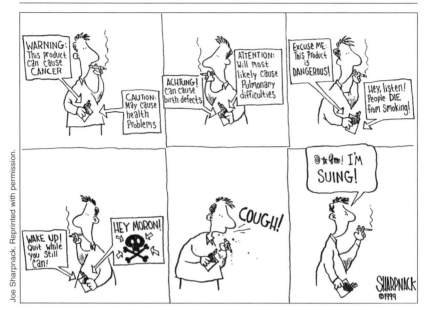

toon figure of Joe Camel and the cowboy images of the
Marlboro Man.

But there is little evidence to support the claim that advertising leads anyone, adults or teens, to smoke. "Repeated statistical analyses have failed to detect a substantial effect on [tobacco] consumption from advertising," writes John E. Calfee of the American Enterprise Institute. Moreover, the claim that advertising causes young people to smoke defies common sense. "Tell a teenager that advertising is the reason he smokes," notes Calfee, "and you will probably convince a teenager that you are out of touch with reality."[2] The reality, as economics professor D.T. Armentano explains, is that "the decision to start using tobacco products is influenced primarily by culture, family, and peer pressure, not corporate advertising."[3]

Tobacco companies do not advertise cigarettes to promote smoking per se, but rather to increase their market share—the popularity of their specific brand. "Critics of the industry have been quick to seize upon studies indicating that teenage smokers disproportionately prefer the most advertised cigarette brands," notes Sullum. "But such research suggests only that advertising has an impact on brand preferences, which the tobacco companies have conceded all along. . . . It is just as plausible to suppose that teenagers pay more attention to cigarette ads after they start smoking."[4]

The "advertising-made-me-smoke" argument is not only specious but also sends a terrible message to teens, in effect telling them that they can blame others for their decision to smoke. Theologian and talk-show host Dennis Prager explains: "It tells them that if they smoke, they do so solely because they have been manipulated by tobacco-company ads . . . that they are helpless when confronted with a billboard for Marlboro cigarettes."[5] Morris E. Chafetz, author of *The Tyranny of Experts: Blowing the Whistle on the Cult of Expertise*, writes: "Such arguments imply that young people are like animals that respond mindlessly to stimuli."[6]

Blaming Addiction

Finally, plaintiffs in tobacco lawsuits have argued that though smokers might choose to start smoking, once they begin they are unable to stop because smoking is so addictive. However, the idea that tobacco companies are to blame for a smoker's addiction is fraught with complications. As psychologist Hans Eysenck explains, "The term 'addiction' has no scientific meaning; it is used in so many different ways that it is almost impossible to attach any meaning for it." For example, various people claim to be addicted not just to drugs, but to sex, overeating, shoplifting, and a variety of other behaviors. How can anyone tell whether a person is addicted to smoking, sex, or eating, or merely enjoys the habit? "There are very good reasons why people continue to smoke," notes Eysenck, "because it has consequences to them that are favourable, agreeable, positive—you don't have to posit a mysterious factor which makes them go on."[7]

Moreover, the claim that it is *impossible* to quit smoking is simply false, as evidenced by the over 46 million former smokers in the United States, most of whom quit cold turkey. "We make entirely too much of the concept of addiction," argues syndicated columnist Mona Charen. "All habits are hard to break. Addiction makes them harder to break. But it does not—as so many seem to assume—make them impossible to break."[8] Patricia Henley, the California recipient of $51.5 million, successfully quit smoking in 1997.

A Return to Individual Responsibility

Each year, millions of Americans take up the habit of smoking. Millions also quit that habit. In each case, the decision to smoke or not to smoke is an individual choice. Neither tobacco companies nor their advertising are responsible for an individual's decision to smoke. All smokers, even those who have become "addicted," are capable of quitting. "The price of freedom in a free society is responsibility for the consequences of one's actions,"[9] writes psychologist and professor Jeffrey A. Schaler. Holding tobacco companies rather than individuals responsible for the consequences of their decisions is simply wrong.

1. Jacob Sullum, "Whose Risk Is It, Anyway?" *New York Times*, February 19, 1999, p. A21.

2. John E. Calfee, "Why the War on Tobacco Will Fail," *Weekly Standard*, July 20, 1998, p. 24.

3. Quoted in Laura K. Egendorf, ed., *Teens at Risk: Opposing Viewpoints*. San Diego: Greenhaven Press, 1997, p. 172.

4. Jacob Sullum, "Cowboys, Camels, and Kids: Does Advertising Turn People into Smokers?" *Reason*, April 1998, www.reason.com/9804/fe.sullum.html.

5. Dennis Prager, "The Soul-Corrupting Anti-Tobacco Crusade," *Weekly Standard*, July 20, 1998, p. 22.

6. Quoted in James D. Torr, ed., *Alcoholism: Current Controversies*. San Diego: Greenhaven Press, 2000, p. 128.

7. Quoted in Judith Hatton, "Smoking and Addiction," *Free Choice*, January/February 1996, http://forest-on-smoking.org.uk/factsheets/aaddict.htm.

8. Quoted in Carol Wekesser, ed., *Smoking: Current Controversies*. San Diego: Greenhaven Press, 1997, p. 77.

9. Quoted in Jeffrey A. Schaler and Magda E. Schaler, eds., *Smoking: Who Has the Right?* Amherst, NY: Prometheus Books, 1998, p. 334.

"Tobacco companies have spent decades deceiving the public about the effects of their cigarettes, and they should be made to pay for it."

Lawsuits Against Tobacco Companies Are Justified

In 1998, the tobacco industry settled out of court with forty-six states that had brought lawsuits against it. The states charged that the tobacco industry had concealed the dangers of cigarette smoking and nicotine addiction and purposely marketed its products to minors. In the 1998 settlement, Big Tobacco agreed to pay the states $206 billion over twenty-five years and to reform its advertising practices. Individuals have also brought claims against the industry, often in class-action lawsuits (cases in which many persons are legally represented as one plaintiff). In June 2000, a Florida jury ordered the tobacco industry to pay $145 billion in punitive damages to a group of seven hundred thousand ex-smokers, on the grounds that the industry deliberately misled smokers about health risks.

These lawsuits have generated headlines around the country. But as *Washington Post* staff writer Joan Biskupic notes, "Lawsuits condemning cigarettes . . . are nothing new. Advocacy groups have campaigned for years against tobacco [companies] . . . , using the courts as a weapon. What is new is that juries are listening."[1]

Turning the Tide Against Big Tobacco

For years, fighting Big Tobacco in court was an almost hope-less battle. Of more than eight hundred claims filed against the tobacco industry between 1954 and 1994, fewer than fifty went to trial, often because the cigarette companies' lawyers would drag out the cases, driving up legal costs so that most plaintiffs could not afford to pursue protracted litigation. Of the fifty cases that did go to trial prior to 1994, the industry lost only three, and two of those were overturned on appeal. Commenting on these four decades, in which Big Tobacco was virtually immune to lawsuits, Edward L. Koven, author of *Smoking: The Story Behind the Maze*, laments, "It is unfortunate in our society that the only industry which produces a con-sumer product that is likely to kill and render human beings seriously ill when used as intended has been so successful in combating challenges within our judicial framework."[2]

Fortunately, the tide is finally turning. "The American legal system may be finally assisting in the exposure of the mer-chants of death,"[3] writes Koven. The courts are at last acknowledging the truth—that "for years, the tobacco indus-try has marketed products that it knew caused serious disease and death. Yet, it intentionally hid this truth from the public, carried out a deceitful campaign to undermine the public's appreciation of these risks, and marketed its addictive prod-ucts to children,"[4] as former surgeon general C. Everett Koop, former FDA director David A. Kessler, and *Journal of the American Medical Association (JAMA)* editor George D. Lundberg state in a *JAMA* editorial.

There are several reasons why the tobacco companies became more vulnerable to litigation in the 1990s. First, the class-action lawsuit allows one law firm to file a case on behalf of thousands of individuals, as in the Florida case. "This strat-egy," writes Koven, "deprives tobacco companies of being able to pursue the normal tactic of forcing plaintiffs to spend huge amounts of money and eventually being forced to withdraw the lawsuits because of lack of funds."[5] In addition, the public's awareness of the addictive nature of smoking has grown since the 1950s, making the tobacco industry's claims that nicotine is not addictive appear increasingly duplicitous. The public's outrage at an industry that has made billions selling sickness and death has also certainly influenced judges and juries—a 1999 *Washington Post* survey found that 59 percent of Americans think the tobacco industry has behaved irresponsibly in selling its products.

The Cigarette Papers

But the definitive proof of Big Tobacco's irresponsible practices came in the form of internal industry documents that were made public in the 1990s. In 1994, more than eight thousand documents were taken from the tobacco giant Brown and Williamson by whistle-blower Merrell Williams (the documents were published in the 1996 book *The Cigarette Papers*). Then in April 1998 the five major tobacco companies produced several thousand more documents in response to subpoenas from the U.S. House of Representatives in the case of *State of Minnesota et al. v. Philip Morris, Inc.*

These documents reveal a decades-long pattern of deception within the tobacco industry. For example, industry documents show that the companies were aware of the link between smoking and lung cancer prior to the first surgeon-general report on the subject in 1964, even though they denied such a link for years. A 1961 report to the Ligget Group states, "There are biologically active materials present in cigarette tobacco. These are cancer causing, cancer promoting, poisonous."[6]

The documents also describe Big Tobacco's deceitful strategy for dealing with studies that linked smoking and disease. In 1954 the industry created the Tobacco Industry Research Committee, later renamed the Council for Tobacco Research (CTR). Ostensibly, its purpose was to research the health effects of cigarettes; in reality CTR worked to convince the

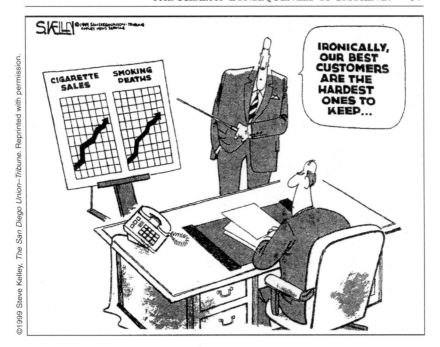

public that the evidence linking cigarettes and lung cancer was "inconclusive." A 1967 policy paper from the organization states, "The smoking of tobacco continues to be one of the subjects requiring study in the lung cancer problem. . . . There can be no promise of a quick answer. The important thing is to keep adding to knowledge until the accumulative facts provide the basis for a sound conclusion."[7] In a 1976 memo titled "Industry Response to the Cigarette Health Controversy," Ernest Pepples, vice president of Brown and Williamson, admitted that the tobacco industry's "research" had just been a public relations ploy: "The significant expenditures on the question of smoking and health have allowed the industry to take a respectable stand along the following lines—'After millions of dollars and over twenty years of research, the question about smoking and health is still open.'"[8]

Manipulating Nicotine Levels to Hook Smokers

The most damning aspect of these industry documents, however, is that they show, beyond a doubt, that as early as the

1960s tobacco companies knew that the nicotine in tobacco was an addictive drug, even though they denied this fact until well into the 1990s. According to a 1969 Philip Morris report, "The primary motive for smoking is to obtain the pharmacological effect of nicotine."[9] A 1963 report by Brown and Williamson vice president Addison Yeaman states, "*Nicotine* is an addictive drug. We are, then, in the business of selling *nicotine*, an addictive drug effective in the release of stress mechanisms." A 1972 R.J. Reynolds memo concludes, "Our industry is . . . based upon design, manufacture and sale of attractive dosage forms of nicotine. . . . Happily for the tobacco industry, nicotine is both habituating and unique."[10]

Even more reprehensible than this deception, however, is the evidence that the tobacco companies artificially raised nicotine concentrations in cigarettes, thus making their deadly product even more addictive. A 1963 Brown and Williamson memo acknowledges "a correlation between consumer acceptance and nicotine level" and reports that "we have a research program in progress to obtain, by genetic means, any level of nicotine desired. . . . Even now we can regulate, fairly precisely, the nicotine and sugar levels to almost any level management might require." A later Brown and Williamson document reports "genetically engineered tobacco delivering more taste/satisfaction . . . achieved through increased nicotine content versus traditional tobaccos."[11]

A Rogue Industry

These industry documents shatter the traditional defenses that tobacco companies have used to shield themselves from lawsuits. For example, the industry often claims that smokers "know the risks" of smoking—but the evidence shows that for decades the industry worked to cast doubt on the link between smoking and lung disease. The tobacco companies also have claimed that people smoke only for "pleasure" or "flavor" and that nicotine is not addictive—but industry documents show that these are flat-out lies.

Big Tobacco should be held legally accountable for its actions. According to the Campaign for Tobacco-Free Kids, tobacco use accounts for roughly $89 billion in public and private health-care costs *each year*. The $209 billion awarded to the states in the 1998 multistate tobacco settlement is actually only a small fraction of the costs that tobacco use has inflicted on society over the decades. Further lawsuits against the industry are also justified. For example, the Department of the Treasury estimates that tobacco use accounts for approximately $20.5 billion in annual federal Medicare expenditures, leading President Bill Clinton to conclude, "The states have been right about this: Taxpayers shouldn't pay for the costs of lung cancer, emphysema, and other smoking-related illnesses; the tobacco companies should."[12] In his February 19, 1999, State of the Union Address the president announced that the Justice Department was preparing a litigation plan to take the tobacco companies to court and use the funds it recovers to strengthen Medicare.

For decades, Big Tobacco has made a profit by selling the instruments of disease and death. As Koop, Kessler, and Lundberg write, "The tobacco makers have shown themselves to be a rogue industry, unwilling to abide by ordinary ethical business standards. . . . [Their] actions are morally reprehensible."[13] It is about time that the justice system holds the industry accountable for its vile behavior. In the end, notes Biskupic, the legal justification for lawsuits against the tobacco industry is pretty simple: "Tobacco companies have spent decades deceiving the public about the effects of their cigarettes, and they should be made to pay for it."[14]

1. Joan Biskupic, "Legislation by Litigation," *Washington Post*, September 3, 1999, p. 6.

2. Edward L. Koven, *Smoking: The Story Behind the Maze*. Commack, NY: Kroshka Books, 1998, p. 97.

3. Koven, *Smoking*, p. 105.

4. C. Everett Koop, David A. Kessler, and George D. Lundberg, "Reinventing American Tobacco Policy," *JAMA*, February 18, 1998, p. 550.

5. Koven, *Smoking*, p. 102.

6. Quoted in David Tannenbaum, "Smoking Guns II: Nicotine Manipulation," *Multinational Monitor*, July/August 1998, p. 25.

7. Quoted in Stanton A. Glantz et al., *The Cigarette Papers*. Berkeley and Los Angeles: University of California Press, 1996, p. 39.

8. Quoted in Glantz, *The Cigarette Papers*, p. 32.

9. Quoted in Campaign for Tobacco-Free Kids, "In the Tobacco Industry's Own Words: Nicotine as a Drug," http://tobaccofreekids.org/research/factsheets/pdf/0009.pdf.

10. Quoted in Tannenbaum, "Smoking Guns II," p. 24.

11. Quoted in Tannenbaum, "Smoking Guns II," p. 24.

12. Quoted in *CQ Researcher*, "Closing in on Tobacco," November 12, 1999, p. 991.

13. Koop, Kessler, and Lundberg, "Reinventing American Tobacco Policy," p. 550.

14. Biskupic, "Legislation by Litigation," p. 6.

"Using the courts to bully [the tobacco industry] in this way is an abuse of the legal process and an evasion of individual responsibility."

Lawsuits Against Tobacco Companies Are Not Justified

The 1990s were witness to a new phenomenon in American politics: legislation by litigation. State governments, seizing on the popular myth that smokers are victims of the tobacco industry, filed lawsuits seeking damages. The states claimed that tobacco companies owed them for the cost of treating smoking-related illnesses. In 1998 the tobacco companies settled out of court, agreeing to pay $209 billion to the states over twenty-five years and to severely restrict their advertising practices.

The regulations set forth in the 1998 multistate tobacco settlement now operate as the law of the land with respect to tobacco advertising. And the settlement effectively put a new cigarette tax into place, since tobacco companies have raised the average price of a pack of cigarettes by approximately 75 cents in order to pay the states their $209 billion. Thus, the settlement has the effect of legislation—legislation that was never voted on by the American people. "Congress has rejected sweeping regulations [on tobacco] because millions of Americans oppose them,"[1] argues a *National Review* editorial.

But the public's voice has been superseded by a legal system out of control.

The 1998 settlement is a travesty of justice, in which public opinion won out over justice. State governments used the courts to extort billions of dollars from an unpopular—but nonetheless legal—industry. Trial lawyers were eager to join in and earn millions of dollars of fees in the process. As *Weekly Standard* editor David Tell notes, "Trial lawyers are more addicted to money than any smoker is to nicotine."[2]

Government Hypocrisy

In court, lawyers representing the states emphasized the deadly nature of cigarette smoke, stressed the addictive nature of nicotine, and trotted out exaggerated statistics on how much lung cancer and emphysema cost state health-care systems. But as syndicated columnist Stephen Chapman pointed out prior to the settlement, "The states involved in the lawsuits are also guilty. If they thought smoking was too costly a vice to indulge, they could have banned it—instead of milking it for billions in tax revenue."[3]

The truth is that the government has no interest in banning cigarettes—not because politicians respect the right of individuals to smoke, but because government revenues from taxing cigarettes are enormous. As of 2000, the federal excise tax on cigarettes was 34 cents per pack, and that is scheduled to increase to 39 cents per pack in 2002. In 1999, the average state excise tax on cigarettes was 39 cents per pack.

Considering that there are millions of smokers in the United States, each buying perhaps hundreds of packs of cigarettes a year, the total government revenue from cigarette sales is in the billions. Even assuming that the "health-care costs of smoking" are as high as antismoking activists claim, "tobacco companies and their customers have more than paid their way,"[4] says Robert A. Levy of the Cato Institute, a libertarian think tank.

Smoking Saves Society Money

But the health-care costs of smoking are not as high as is often claimed. Estimates of the health-care costs of smoking simply tally the costs of treating lung cancer, emphysema, and so forth. They are inflated because they ignore the fact that if all the smokers in America had never lit a single cigarette, they would eventually die anyway. The actual "health-care cost of smoking" is not simply the cost of treating smoking-related diseases, but the *difference* between treating smoking-related diseases and all the "normal" diseases that nonsmokers die from: heart disease, pneumonia, Alzheimer's disease, and so forth. No one has ever proven in court that this *net* cost is significant.

Instead, a significant argument can be made that smoking actually saves the government money—and that therefore the entire basis for the states' lawsuits against the tobacco industry is false. Smokers' premature deaths mean that the government spends less money on smokers' retirement payments and nursing home care. And tallying the escalating medical costs associated with old age, smokers' health-care bills are, over a lifetime, lower than nonsmokers'. These facts led a 1997 study in the *New England Journal of Medicine* to conclude, "If people stopped smoking, there would be savings in health care costs, but only in the short term. Eventually, smoking cessation would lead to increased health care costs."[5]

Punishing Smokers, Not the Tobacco Industry

Antismoking zealots don't seem to mind that the health-care arguments surrounding their case are not credible: Regardless of the exact costs smoking has imposed on the states, they argue, the tobacco industry should be punished for its irresponsible marketing practices. But the wave of lawsuits against the industry certainly hasn't harmed the people who, for example, designed the Joe Camel ad campaign or raised nicotine levels in cigarettes. "Not one wrongdoer . . . has ever been significantly impoverished or otherwise punished by a tobacco lawsuit," notes Stuart Taylor Jr. of the *National Journal.* "Rather, the mass of litigation . . . quite clearly operates not as a punishment, but as a national tax that no representative body ever sought to impose."[6]

The $209 billion the tobacco companies were forced to pay to the states in 1998 is not coming from the pockets of Big Tobacco executives. Rather than losing profits and going out of business, cigarette companies have simply raised cigarette prices. Writing in July 2000, Taylor notes that smokers "are already paying an average of $2.81 for a pack of coffin nails— a 37 percent increase since November 1998 [when the tobacco settlement was announced]."[7] It is smokers, not tobacco companies, who are footing the bill for anti-tobacco lawsuits. This is ironic given that one supposed purpose of the lawsuits was to "protect" smokers.

Critics claim that the $209 billion settlement the tobacco companies were required to pay to the states is, in effect, paid for by smokers in the form of raised cigarette prices.

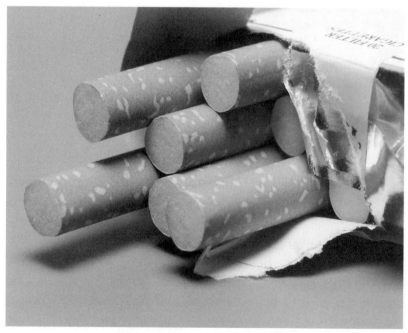

The way to punish misconduct by tobacco executives is to sue them personally or punish them criminally. But although the federal government has been investigating the tobacco industry since the mid-1990s, there has not been a single indictment of a tobacco company or industry executive.

Little Benefit to Public Health

Of course, antismoking activists can ignore the fact that smokers are footing the bill for the $209 billion the states are set to receive. In their eyes, it doesn't matter that the settlement amounts to legalized mugging, as long as the money will help reduce smoking. But it is evident that the lawsuit will do little to reduce youth smoking or otherwise improve public health. "Now that the loot is rolling in from the multistate settlement [in early 2000]," writes Levy, "we know that kids' welfare is far down the list of priorities. In Los Angeles the money will be used to improve sidewalks; in Michigan it'll allow a cut in college tuition; in North Dakota flood control gets the nod. In only a handful of states is funding tobacco control programs significantly beyond presettlement levels."[8]

A Dangerous Precedent

While the states' lawsuits against the industry have done little to help smokers, they have seriously harmed the legal system. As Gayle M.B. Hanson, a writer for *Insight on the News* magazine, warns, the tobacco lawsuits "set a dangerous precedent that could result in a massive wave of lawsuits targeted at other industries that are perceived to be politically incorrect or cause public harm."[9] For example, in the wake of tobacco lawsuits, suits have been brought against gun manufacturers for causing crime. In February 1999, just months after the multistate settlement was announced, a Brooklyn jury ruled that gun makers should pay damages because some of their firearms are used by criminals.

The arguments used against cigarettes are applicable to all sorts of "unhealthy" items: Beer and liquor companies—perhaps even fast-food restaurants!—could also be subject to litigation. "As I understand it," explains *Washington Post* editor Fred Barbash, "fat, when used as intended, causes heart disease, which actually kills more people than smoking."[10] And if tobacco advertising causes people to smoke, then surely fast-food advertising causes people to eat unhealthy quantities of fat. "What . . . is the substantive difference," asks Hanson, "between Ronald McDonald's ubiquitous pleas to imbibe ever more fat-laden burgers and fries and Joe Camel's exhortation to light up?"[11]

Could lawsuits against McDonald's, followed by an out-of-court settlement that raises the price of cheeseburgers and restricts "fat advertising," be around the corner? The zealotry of the antismoking crusade could easily be extended to ludicrous proportions. For precisely these reasons psychology professor Jeffrey A. Schaler warns: "The increasing attempt to hold tobacco companies responsible for the consequences of smoking behavior poses a greater threat to liberty in a free society than nicotine ever could."[12]

The United States vs. Big Tobacco?

"Using the courts to bully industries in this way is an abuse of the legal process and an evasion of individual responsibility,"[13] states an *Economist* writer. But that's not going to stop the federal government. In 1999 President Clinton announced that, like the states, the federal government is going to sue the tobacco industry for health-care costs. Just like the state lawsuits, this federal lawsuit will be based on false premises; its costs will be borne by smokers, not the tobacco companies; it will do little to reduce smoking; and it will set a dangerous legal precedent. In the rush to condemn Big Tobacco, even the president has lost sight of the fact that public policy should not be decided by lawsuit.

1. *National Review*, "Public Policy: Legal Muggings," April 17, 2000.

2. David Tell, "A New Direction on the Tobacco Road," *Weekly Standard*, May 5, 1997, p. 9.

3. Quoted in Mary E. Williams and Tamara L. Roleff, eds., *Tobacco and Smoking: Opposing Viewpoints*. San Diego: Greenhaven Press, 1998, p. 169.

4. Robert A. Levy, "The Tobacco Deal: Myths and Misconceptions," *Freeman*, January 1998, p. 20.

5. Jan J. Barendregt, Luc Bonneux, and Paul J. van der Maas, "The Health Care Costs of Smoking," *New England Journal of Medicine*, October 9, 1997, p. 1,052.

6. Stuart Taylor Jr., "Tobacco Lawsuits: Taxing the Victims to Enrich the Lawyers," *National Journal*, July 29, 2000.

7. Taylor, "Tobacco Lawsuits."

8. Robert A. Levy, "When Theft Masquerades as Law," *Cato Policy Report*, March/April 2000, p. 9.

9. Gayle M.B. Hanson, "Tobacco and Liberty," *Insight on the News*, March 16, 1998, p. 9.

10. Fred Barbash, "Warning: Zealotry May Be Hazardous to Your Health," *Washington Post*, April 27, 1998, p. 23.

11. Hanson, "Tobacco and Liberty," p. 11.

12. Quoted in Jeffrey A. Schaler and Magda E. Schaler, eds., *Smoking: Who Has the Right?* Amherst, NY: Prometheus Books, 1998, p. 332.

13. *Economist*, "When Lawsuits Make Policy," November 21, 1998.

CHAPTER 3

Should the Government Increase Efforts to Reduce Smoking?

"Comprehensive national tobacco control legislation will move us all toward a healthier America."

The Government Should Increase Efforts to Reduce Smoking

Tobacco use, particularly smoking, remains the number one cause of preventable disease and death in the United States. In the 1990s, growing awareness of the hazards of smoking, combined with evidence of the tobacco industry's irresponsible behavior in promoting smoking and covering up its dangers, led to numerous lawsuits against the industry. However, it is clear that these lawsuits are an incomplete solution to the problem of smoking in America. For example, despite the restrictions the industry agreed to in the 1998 multistate tobacco settlement, cigarette companies are still free to advertise in youth-oriented magazines; children and teens are still able to purchase cigarettes in vending machines; and smoking is still permitted in public buildings in many states. It is clear that to properly serve public health, the United States must adopt a comprehensive, nationwide tobacco control plan.

Allow the Food and Drug Administration to Regulate Tobacco

The best way to insure appropriate regulation of tobacco products would be to grant the Food and Drug Administration

(FDA) authority to regulate tobacco. "We can't hide from the fact that nicotine is a drug," says former FDA chairman David A. Kessler. "The nation's most important consumer protection agency that regulates all other addictive drugs should regulate this drug."[1] Moreover, as Bill Novelli, president of the Campaign for Tobacco-Free Kids, explains:

> FDA is the only government agency that can provide comprehensive oversight of all aspects of tobacco-product development and marketing, including the companies' use of dangerous chemical additives, their nicotine manipulation and their advertising and promotional efforts to attract kids. Compared to Congress or the state legislatures, the FDA also has the ability to modify its regulations swiftly to counteract changes in tobacco-industry tactics . . . and is less likely to be corrupted or impeded by tobacco-company money and influence.[2]

Unfortunately, the Supreme Court ruled in April 2000 that, under current law, the FDA lacks the authority to regulate tobacco. It is therefore up to Congress to change the law and provide the FDA with the authority it needs to regulate tobacco, so that cigarettes will be subject to the same labeling, product-safety, and consumer-protection laws as other consumer products.

Raise Cigarette Prices

While Congress debates FDA regulation of tobacco, lawmakers should immediately take another simple step to significantly reduce smoking in the United States: raise excise taxes on tobacco. As a 2000 report from the surgeon general notes, "Raising tobacco excise taxes is widely regarded as one of the most effective tobacco prevention and control strategies."[3] A study published in the September 2000 issue of *Preventive Medicine* predicts that if cigarette taxes are raised by $1 per pack, more than 2.3 million fewer Americans will die prematurely from smoking-related diseases in the next forty years; an increase of only 20 cents per pack would save over a million lives in the next four decades.

The United States would do well to follow the example of other industrialized nations in this regard. According to physician Thomas Houston and nurse Nancy J. Kaufman, "Tobacco excise taxes in the United States are comparatively low. For example, taxes in Denmark, the United Kingdom, and India make up about 80% of the retail price. In the United States, taxes are less than 40% of the total retail price."[4] "Canada slapped a heavy user fee on cigarettes from 1981 to 1992," notes John J. Lynch, president of the American Cancer Society's mid-Atlantic division. "The result? A 38 percent downturn in smoking overall and a 60 percent decline in youth smoking."[5]

"Smokers' rights" groups claim that raising taxes on cigarettes harms lower-income smokers. On the contrary: It helps them. As Lynch explains, "Faced with higher cigarette prices, more nonsmokers will choose not to start, and more smokers will choose to cut back or even quit—especially kids. These choices are highly beneficial to those who make them, their loved ones, and to society."[6]

Ban Tobacco Advertising

Another way to reduce smoking is to ban tobacco advertising. A partial ban—such as that currently prohibiting tobacco advertising on television and radio—has little effect because tobacco companies simply transfer their vast resources to other types of promotion, such as print media. The United States should follow Europe's example. The European Union has voted that all tobacco advertising—through magazines, newspapers, radio, television, billboards, and event sponsorship—be banned by 2006.

Tobacco companies sometimes claim that the First Amendment—which protects the right of free speech—makes such an advertising ban unconstitutional. But the Supreme

Court ruled in a landmark 1980 decision that commercial speech (advertising) is not subject to the same First Amendment protections as other types of speech. The Court reasoned that certain types of commercial speech may be regulated in the public interest. A ban on tobacco advertising certainly fits that requirement. Moreover, as Larry C. White, the author of *Merchants of Death: The American Tobacco Industry*, puts it, "Can anyone seriously believe that the First Amendment was intended to protect the right of a powerful industry to use highly sophisticated methods of mass persuasion in order to sell a deadly and addictive product?"[7]

Protect the Public from Secondhand Smoke

Comprehensive tobacco control legislation must also recognize that cigarette smoke harms nonsmokers, too. A 1997 report from the California Environmental Protection Agency estimates that, each year, environmental tobacco smoke (ETS) causes three thousand deaths due to lung cancer, as well as over thirty-five thousand deaths due to ischemic heart disease. Clearly the government has a responsibility to protect nonsmokers from the harmful effects of this type of air pollution, yet many states still permit smoking in public buildings. "Smoking should be banned in all work sites and in all places of public assembly, especially those in places in which children are present,"[8] concludes a report to Congress from the Advisory Committee on Tobacco Policy and Public Health.

"Most people spend about 90% of their time in 2 'microenvironments': home and work," notes physician Ronald M. Davis. "Thus, populations at greater risk of harm from ETS are those who live with smokers and those who work where smoking is allowed."[9] Government cannot ban smoking in private homes, but government can—and should—pass laws to ensure the safety of individuals in the workplace. Restaurants, bars, and casinos are all venues in which ETS concentrations are relatively high. States should ban smoking in these types of establishments, but most have not. As of

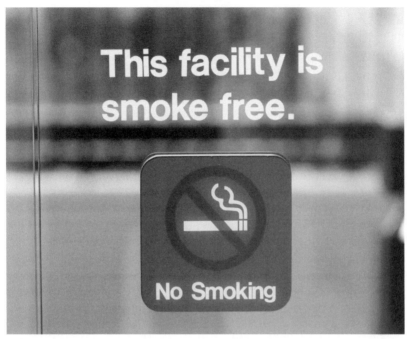

While smoking is not permitted in many workplaces and public buildings, it is often allowed in restaurants, bars, and casinos, a policy that some experts believe is a danger to public health.

September 2000, only California has passed a law to protect workers by banning smoking in bars. Federal legislation would minimize the hazards of ETS for both workers and the general public.

State Tobacco Prevention Efforts

These are the key elements of tobacco control, but a truly comprehensive governmental response to smoking aims to "change the whole social norm about tobacco,"[10] as Colleen Stevens, chief of California's antismoking media campaign, puts it. To this end, government should sponsor a variety of programs: antismoking media campaigns, community and school-based education programs, and programs that help smokers quit.

Several states have raised cigarette taxes and used the resulting revenue to fund exactly these types of tobacco prevention programs. The Campaign for Tobacco-Free Kids reports that cigarette consumption in California, which instituted a comprehensive tobacco prevention program in 1988, has declined by 38 percent, compared with a national average of 16 percent over the same time period. Massachusetts began a similar program in 1992, and has seen a decrease in cigarette consumption of 30 percent. These states' successes indicate that antismoking education efforts, in combination with the measures listed above, could lead to unprecedented declines in smoking nationwide.

Responding to "Smokers' Rights" Arguments

Some people have claimed that tobacco control efforts infringe on an individual's "right to smoke." This is an exaggeration: No one is proposing that tobacco use be made illegal, or that adults shouldn't be allowed to smoke in areas where it will not harm others.

An even greater exaggeration made by tobacco companies is that regulations on tobacco might lead to regulations on other unhealthy products, such as foods that are high in fat. It is a measure of tobacco industry deceit to compare *taking a poison* to eating food! The fact is that fat, and even other potentially harmful substances such as alcohol, are only dangerous when taken in excess. Tobacco is the only product that is harmful *when used as intended.*

Toward a Healthier America

"Comprehensive national tobacco control legislation will move us all toward a healthier America," writes Lynch. "There are no losers except the tobacco companies. And they deserve to lose because they've caused so much illness and death by suppressing what they know about the dangers of their products."[11] For decades the tobacco industry has made a profit selling a product that kills an estimated four hundred thousand Americans each year, and the U.S. government has done shamefully little about it. But it's not too late to help save America's youth. The time for comprehensive tobacco control is now.

1. David A. Kessler, "Time to Act on Cigarettes," *Washington Post*, April 10, 2000, p. 27.

2. Bill Novelli, "Should the FDA Assume Regulatory Power over Tobacco Products? Yes: An Agency Free from Political Influence Is Situated to Rein in This Rogue Industry," *Insight on the News*, May 10, 1999, p. 24.

3. Centers for Disease Control and Prevention, "Reducing Tobacco Use: A Report of the Surgeon General: At-a-Glance," 2000, www.cdc.gov/tobacco/sgr_tobacco_pdf/aag2cpy.pdf.

4. Thomas Houston and Nancy J. Kaufman, "Tobacco Control in the 21st Century," *JAMA*, August 9, 2000, p. 752.

5. John J. Lynch, "Do We Need a Tobacco Bill? Emphatically Yes, and Now," *World & I*, July 1998, p. 73.

6. Lynch, "Do We Need a Tobacco Bill?" p. 72.

7. Larry C. White, "Is Cigarette Advertising Protected by the First Amendment? No," *Priorities*, vol. 5, no. 3, 1993, www.acsh.org/publications/priorities/0503/pcpno.html.

8. Advisory Committee on Tobacco Policy and Public Health, "Summary of the Major Recommendations of the Task Force on Environmental Tobacco Smoke," 1997, www.lungusa.org/tobacco/smkkoop.html.

9. Ronald M. Davis, "Exposure to Environmental Tobacco Smoke: Identifying and Protecting Those at Risk," *JAMA*, December 9, 1998, p. 1,947.

10. Quoted in Ira Teinowitz, "Just Take the Money and Run (the Ads)," *Washington Post*, December 14, 1998, p. 21.

11. Lynch, "Do We Need a Tobacco Bill?" p. 74.

"The antismoking movement is about making people healthier, even if that means taking away their freedom."

The Government Should Respect Smokers' Rights

Antismoking activists are quick to use the phrase "smoking kills." This is an oversimplification. While it is true that *some* smokers die from diseases such as lung cancer and emphysema that *may have been* caused by smoking, it is certainly not true that smoking kills all smokers. Estimates of the proportion of smokers who die from smoking-related illnesses range from about one-third to about one-half.

Smoking is a risky activity, not necessarily a deadly one. And adults in a free society have the right to engage in risky activities if they so choose. Thus adults have a right to smoke—or rather, the government has no right to prohibit them from smoking. "Just because some people make what most people consider to be the wrong choices does not mean government should do the choosing," writes Jon Saunders, a research associate at the Pope Center for Higher Education Reform. "Allowing foolish choices is far wiser than sacrificing the freedom to choose. As Gandhi said, 'Freedom is not worth having if it does not connote freedom to err.'"[1]

Specious Arguments

Of course, antismoking advocates pretend that "tobacco control" initiatives are not intended to encroach on the rights of adults. They routinely insist that antismoking legislation is necessary to protect children. But all fifty states have laws against cigarette sales to minors; these laws can and should be more strongly enforced. And schools can and should teach children about the dangers of smoking. These measures do not impinge on the free choices of adults. But antismoking crusaders want to go much further.

Not only must children be protected, they argue, but adults must be protected from the dangers of secondhand smoke, or environmental tobacco smoke (ETS). According to this view, the dangers of ETS justify all sorts of bans on smoking—in the workplace, in government buildings, in restaurants, even in bars and casinos!

But where is the evidence that ETS poses a significant health hazard to nonsmokers? Elizabeth M. Whelan, president of the American Council on Science and Health, an organization that supports tobacco control, concedes, "The role of ETS in the development of chronic diseases like cancer and heart disease is uncertain and controversial."[2] In 1998 the World Health Organization (WHO) concluded a seven-year study of 650 lung cancer patients and 1,546 healthy people. The study examined people who were married to smokers, worked with smokers, and grew up with smokers and found that their risk of lung cancer was not significantly higher than anyone else's. Yet these findings received little attention in the American press, largely because the anti-tobacco crusade has brainwashed most Americans into flatly accepting the preposterous notion that being in a room with smokers is just as dangerous as smoking itself.

The antismoking movement is not about protecting children, nor is it about secondhand smoke. As a 2000 report by the surgeon general is bluntly titled, it is about "Reducing

Tobacco Use." The antismoking movement is about making people healthier, even if that means taking away their freedom.

Cigarette Taxes: A Form of Social Control

For example, one of the favorite goals of tobacco control advocates is to raise taxes on cigarettes. What they rarely acknowledge is that cigarette taxes are essentially taxes on the poor. As columnist Robert J. Samuelson explains in *Newsweek*, "Smokers have low incomes. Only 20 percent of cigarette taxes are paid by those with incomes over $50,000; 34 percent are paid by those with incomes under $20,000 and 19 percent by those with incomes between $20,000 and $30,000."[3] Cigarette taxes create a situation in which only the rich, who can afford the extra costs, are able to smoke. This protects neither children nor nonsmokers; all it does is artificially raise the price of a product that all adults should be allowed to freely enjoy.

Cigarette taxation is, quite simply, a form of social control—an attempt by a high-minded government elite to shape the behavior of the masses "for their own good." Government laws that make cigarettes unaffordable are no different than laws that would make cigarettes illegal.

Bans on Advertising: A Violation of the First Amendment

The regulation of cigarette advertising is another way the government tries to control the choices of adults, by limiting their access to information. Tobacco advertising is banned on television and radio in the United States. Europe has voted to ban all tobacco advertising by 2006, and antismoking groups in the United States are pushing for the same restrictions.

Ironically, bans on advertising actually help the established tobacco companies, by making it almost impossible for new, competing cigarette brands—even ones that might be safer in terms of tar and nicotine content—to be successful. But far worse than this practical downside to the bans is the chilling effect they have on free speech. To understand why, writes Robert Peck of the American Civil Liberties Union, "Put aside the fact that tobacco is the subject of the advertisement. Imagine if a state banned ads that promoted abortion services or any other controversial products. . . . Surely, it becomes more obvious that this is an infringement on our free-speech rights." Peck concludes, "The battle to improve public health should not require us to trample upon our vibrant free-speech tradition."[4]

The Rise of the Nanny State

Americans seem to have lost sight of the fact that it is not the government's job to make sure that people always make the "right" decisions about their health. Moreover, it is a threat to individual liberty when the government coerces people into making healthy choices. For example, psychology professor Jeffrey A. Schaler asks:

> If government has the power to protect people from making choices that involve relatively high risks, why stop at tobacco consumption? What about skiing, mountain climbing, hang gliding, drinking alcohol, and working long hours? Are the risks "too high"? By whose standard? . . . If the government is going to enact coercive measures that arbitrarily restrict the liberties and trample on the rights of smokers, where will employment of this restrictive power end?[5]

Indeed, "a government empowered to maximize health is a totalitarian government,"[6] as Jacob Sullum concludes in his book *For Your Own Good: The Anti-Smoking Crusade and the Tyranny of Public Health.*

A New Prohibition?

The arguments against tobacco control laws and the antismoking crusade in general are not just ideological. In the 1920s, the temperance movement succeeded in passing the Eighteenth Amendment, which virtually outlawed the manufacture and sale of alcohol in the United States. The result was widespread bootlegging of alcohol and the rise of organized crime. Could America be headed for a similar disaster over tobacco?

There are many parallels between the temperance movement and the antismoking crusade. For example, drinking levels declined well before Prohibition was enacted, just as modern smoking rates have been falling for decades. In addition, as author Mark Lender notes, "Temperance zealots insisted that all drinking led to addiction. This was obvious nonsense, and the public ultimately called them on it. Similarly, many smokers may find it hard to quit, but millions have quit. Exaggerated claims of addiction are the rhetoric of a movement determined on victory at all costs."[7]

Demonizing Smokers

Just as temperance activists railed against "demon rum" in the 1920s, so too do anti-tobacco advocates criticize smoking as evil. The smoking habit is becoming increasingly unpopular, and many people consider it a rude and offensive behavior. But Americans' generally low opinion of smoking does not justify the tobacco control laws that "public health" activists propose. "Citizens in a free society . . . should never confuse their right to disdain rudeness with the government's ability to outlaw it,"[8] writes Saunders.

"The hallmark of a free nation is whether it safeguards the rights of its least popular citizens," writes Robert A. Levy of the Cato Institute. "When it comes to tobacco, we have failed that test."[9]

1. Jon Saunders, "The Tyranny of the Proper," *Ideas on Liberty*, December 1998, www.fee.org/freeman/98/9812/happiness.html.

2. Elizabeth M. Whelan, "Warning: Overstating the Case Against Secondhand Smoke Is Unnecessary—and Harmful to Public Health Policy," American Council on Science and Health editorial, August 1, 2000, www.acsh.org/press/editorials/warning080100.html.

3. Robert J. Samuelson, "The Amazing Smoke Screen," *Newsweek*, November 30, 1998, p. 47.

4. Robert Peck, "Is Cigarette Advertising Protected by the First Amendment? Yes," *Priorities*, vol. 5, no.3, 1993, www.acsh.org/publications.priorities/0503/pcpyes.html.

5. Quoted in Jeffrey A. Schaler and Magda E. Schaler, eds., *Smoking: Who Has the Right?* Amherst, NY: Prometheus Books, 1998, p. 301.

6. Quoted in James D. Torr, ed., *Health Care: Opposing Viewpoints*. San Diego: Greenhaven Press, 2000, p. 151.

7. Mark Lender, "Born Again: The Resurgence of American Prohibition," *Ideas on Liberty*, March 1996, www.fee.org/freeman/96/9604/lender.html.

8. Saunders, "The Tyranny of the Proper."

9. Robert A. Levy, "The Tobacco Deal: Myths and Misconceptions," *Freeman*, January 1998, p. 19.

STUDY QUESTIONS

Chapter 1

1. After reading Viewpoints 1 and 2, do you feel that tobacco control advocates have exaggerated the health threat of smoking? If so, how?

2. Consider the sources of the information in Viewpoints 1 and 2. In Viewpoint 1, most of the data on smoking and health are attributed to government organizations, whereas in Viewpoint 2 much of the quoted material is from independent researchers. How does this affect your opinion of the two viewpoints?

3. Viewpoint 1 argues that smoking is an addiction while Viewpoint 2 argues that it is merely "a bad habit." What evidence is provided to support these two claims, and which do you find most persuasive?

4. Viewpoint 4 argues that individuals do not develop smoking-related diseases as teens, so therefore smoking is not a youth issue. Do you accept this argument? Why or why not?

5. Viewpoints 3 and 4 offer opposing views on whether antismoking campaigns targeted at teens are effective or not. In your own experience, how have school-, community-, or advertising-based antismoking programs influenced your views on smoking?

Chapter 2

1. After reading Viewpoints 1 and 2, do you think individual choice or tobacco advertising is the main reason people decide to smoke? Do you think individual choice or nicotine addiction is the main reason people *continue* to smoke? Explain your answers, using evidence from the viewpoints.

2. Viewpoint 1 argues that virtually all smokers know the dangers of tobacco use. Do you agree with this claim? What evidence is provided in the viewpoint to support it?

3. Viewpoint 2 argues that tobacco advertising is intended to hook young people on smoking. Do you feel that the Marlboro Man or other types of cigarette ads are aimed at teens? Why or why not?

4. In your opinion, should cigarette companies be held partially liable for smoking-related diseases such as lung cancer? How does Viewpoint 3, which argues that cigarette companies have

behaved irresponsibly in the past, affect your opinion on this issue?

5. Review Viewpoint 4 and list its main criticisms of lawsuits against the tobacco industry. Which of these do you find most persuasive, and why?

Chapter 3

1. Viewpoint 1 lists several types of tobacco control measures, including taxes on cigarettes, bans on tobacco advertising, restrictions on smoking in public places, and antismoking educational campaigns. Based on the viewpoints, which of these do you think is most effective? Explain.

2. Do you agree with the Viewpoint 2 claim that individuals have a right to smoke? If not, why not? If so, can you think of reasons why government restrictions on smoking might nevertheless be justified?

3. Viewpoint 2 maintains that the arguments used to justify restrictions and taxes on smoking could be used to justify restrictions on other risky activities, such as skydiving. Do you find this argument convincing? Explain your answer.

APPENDIX A

Facts About Smoking

The Health Effects of Smoking

According to the Centers for Disease Control and Prevention (CDC):

- Smoking can cause a variety of cancers, including cancer of the lung, larynx, oral cavity, esophagus, pancreas, bladder, kidney, stomach, and cervix, as well as leukemia.
- Other smoking-related diseases include hypertension, heart disease, stroke, pneumonia, bronchitis, and emphysema.
- Each year, more than 400,000 Americans die from smoking-related diseases—more than 276,000 men and 142,000 women a year.
- On average, smokers die nearly seven years earlier than non-smokers.
- Men who smoke increase their risk of death from lung cancer by more than 22 times and from bronchitis and emphysema by nearly 10 times. Women who smoke increase their risk of dying from lung cancer by nearly 12 times and their risk of dying from bronchitis and emphysema by more than 10 times.
- Smoking triples the risk of dying from heart disease among middle-aged men and women.

The Prevalence of Adult Smoking

According to the CDC, as of 1997:

- An estimated 48 million (24.7 percent) U.S. adults age 18 years were current smokers—27.6 percent of men and 22.1 percent of women.
- Smoking prevalence was higher among American Indians/Alaska Natives (34 percent), African Americans (26.7 percent), and whites (25.3 percent) than among Hispanics (20.4 percent) and Asian/Pacific Islanders (16.9 percent).
- Smoking prevalence was higher among adults living below the poverty level (33 percent) than those living at or above the poverty level (24.6 percent).
- An estimated 44 million adults (25.1 million men and 19.2 million women) are former smokers. Of the current everyday adult smokers in 1997, approximately 16 million quit smoking for at least one day during the last year.

- The states with the highest current smoking prevalences among adults were Kentucky (30.8 percent), Missouri (28.7 percent), Arkansas (28.5 percent), Nevada (27.7 percent), and West Virginia (27.4 percent).
- The lowest smoking prevalence rates among adults were found in Utah (13.7 percent), followed by California (18.4 percent), Hawaii (18.6 percent), the District of Columbia (18.8 percent), and Idaho (19.9 percent).

The Prevalence of Youth Smoking

According to a 1999 study by the CDC:
- Smoking among ninth- through twelfth-grade students rose from 34.8% in 1995 to 36.4% in 1997, and fell to 34.8% in 1999.
- Approximately one in eight (12.8 percent) middle school students reported using some form of tobacco in the past month.
- Current cigarette use among middle school students was 9.2 percent—9.6 percent for boys and 8.8 percent for girls.
- Approximately 80% of adult smokers started smoking before the age of 18.
- Eighty-six percent of youth smokers prefer the three most heavily advertised brands—Marlboro, Camel, and Newport.

Federal and State Laws on Smoking

Warning labels. The federal government mandates health warning labels on cigarette packages.

Restrictions on advertising. The federal government bans cigarette advertisements on television and radio, and thirteen states legally restrict the advertising and promotion of tobacco products.

Excise taxes. As of 2000, the federal excise tax on cigarettes was 34 cents per pack; it is scheduled to increase to 39 cents per pack in 2002. All states impose an excise tax on cigarettes. As of December 31, 1998, the average tax was 38.9 cents per pack and ranged from 2.5 cents per pack in Virginia to $1 per pack in Alaska and Hawaii.

Smoking in public places. Twenty states limit smoking in private worksites; 41 limit smoking in state government worksites. Thirty states have laws that restrict smoking in restaurants. Twenty-eight states and the District of Columbia have laws that limit smoking in commercial day care centers.

Cigarette sales to minors. All states prohibit the sale of tobacco products to minors. However, only 19 states ban cigarette vending machines in areas accessible to minors.

Appendix B

Related Documents

Document 1: A Frank Statement to Cigarette Smokers

In January 1954, in response to growing numbers of medical reports linking smoking with lung cancer, the tobacco industry ran a full-page advertisement in magazines and newspapers nationwide. In it, the tobacco industry questioned the validity of studies linking cigarettes with cancer, but promised to aid research on the subject with the formation of the Tobacco Industry Research Committee, later renamed the Center for Tobacco Research. A banner at the top of the ad read "A Frank Statement to Cigarette Smokers," and it was signed by heads of 14 tobacco companies. The text of the advertisement is reprinted below.

Recent reports on experiments with mice have given wide publicity to a theory that cigarette smoking is in some way linked with lung cancer in human beings.

Although conducted by doctors of professional standing, these experiments are not regarded as conclusive in the field of cancer research. However, we do not believe that any serious medical research, even though its results are inconclusive, should be disregarded or lightly dismissed.

At the same time, we feel it is in the public interest to call attention to the fact that eminent doctors and research scientists have publicly questioned the claimed significance of these experiments.

Distinguished authorities point out:

1. **That medical research of recent years indicates many possible causes of lung cancer.**
2. **That there is no agreement among the authorities regarding what the cause is.**
3. **That there is no proof that cigarette smoking is one of the causes.**
4. **That statistics purporting to link cigarette smoking with the disease could apply with equal force to any one of many other aspects of modern life. Indeed the validity of the statistics themselves is questioned by numerous scientists.**

We accept an interest in people's health as a basic responsibility, paramount to every other consideration in our business.

We believe the products we make are not injurious to health.

We always have and always will cooperate closely with those whose task it is to safeguard the public health.

For more than 300 years tobacco has given solace, relaxation, and enjoyment to mankind. At one time or another during those years critics have held it responsible for practically every disease of the human body. One by one these charges have been abandoned for lack of evidence.

Regardless of the record of the past, the fact that cigarette smoking today should even be suspected as a cause of serious disease is a matter of deep concern to us.

Many people have asked us what we are doing to meet the public's concern aroused by the recent reports. Here is the answer:

• **We are pledging aid and assistance to the research effort into all phases of tobacco use and health. The joint financial aid will of course be in addition to what is already being contributed by individual companies.**

• **For this purpose we are establishing a joint industry group consisting initially of the undersigned. This group will be known as TOBACCO INDUSTRY RESEARCH COMMITTEE.**

• **In charge of the research activities of the Committee will be a scientist of unimpeachable integrity and national repute. In addition there will be an Advisory Board of scientists disinterested in the cigarette industry. A group of distinguished men from medicine, science, and education will be invited to serve on this Board. These scientists will advise the Committee on its research activities.**

This statement is being issued because we believe the people are entitled to know where we stand on this matter and what we intend to do about it.

Tobacco Industry Research Committee, "A Frank Statement to Smokers," January 1954.

Document 2: The 1964 Surgeon General's Report on Smoking and Health

In 1964 Surgeon General Luther Terry issued the first official statement by the U.S. government linking cigarette smoking and lung cancer. The report's release marked the beginning of the modern tobacco control movement. In the portion excerpted below, the report's major findings on the links between smoking and disease are summarized.

Since the turn of the century, scientists have become increasingly interested in the effects of tobacco on health. Only within the past few decades, however, has a broad experimental and clinical approach to the subject been manifest; within this period the most extensive and definitive studies have been undertaken since 1950.

Few medical questions have stirred such public interest or created more scientific debate than the tobacco-health controversy. The interrelationships of smoking and health undoubtedly are complex. The subject does not lend itself to easy answers. Nevertheless, it has been increasingly apparent that answers must be found. . . .

Accordingly, I appointed a committee, drawn from all the pertinent scientific disciplines, to review and evaluate both this new and older data and, if possible, to reach some definitive conclusions on the relationship between smoking and health in general. The results of the Committee's study and evaluation are contained in this Report. . . .

The Effects of Smoking: Principal Findings

Cigarette smoking is associated with a 70 percent increase in the age-specific death rates of males. The total number of excess deaths causally related to cigarette smoking in the U.S. population cannot be accurately estimated. In view of the continuing and mounting evidence from many sources, it is the judgment of the Committee that cigarette smoking contributes substantially to mortality from certain specific diseases and to the overall death rate.

Lung Cancer. Cigarette smoking is causally related to lung cancer in men; the magnitude of the effect of cigarette smoking far outweighs all other factors. The data for women, though less extensive, point in the same direction.

The risk of developing lung cancer increases with duration of smoking and the number of cigarettes smoked per day, and is diminished by discontinuing smoking. In comparison with non-smokers, average male smokers of cigarettes have approximately a 9- to 10-fold risk of developing lung cancer and heavy smokers at least a 20-fold risk.

The risk of developing cancer of the lung for the combined group of pipe smokers, cigar smokers, and pipe and cigar smokers is greater than for non-smokers, but much less than for cigarette smokers.

Cigarette smoking is much more important than occupational exposures in the causation of lung cancer in the general population.

Chronic Bronchitis and Emphysema. Cigarette smoking is the most important of the causes of chronic bronchitis in the United States, and increases the risk of dying from chronic bronchitis and emphysema. A relationship exists between cigarette smoking and emphysema but it has not been established that the relationship is causal. Studies demonstrate that fatalities from this disease are infrequent among non-smokers.

For the bulk of the population of the United States, the relative importance of cigarette smoking as a cause of chronic broncho-pulmonary disease is much greater than atmospheric pollution or occupational exposures.

Cardiovascular Diseases. It is established that male cigarette smokers have a higher death rate from coronary artery disease than non-smoking males. Although the causative role of cigarette smoking in deaths from coronary disease is not proven, the Committee considers it more prudent from the public health viewpoint to assume that the established association has causative meaning than to suspend judgment until no uncertainty remains.

Although a causal relationship has not been established, higher mortality of cigarette smokers is associated with many other cardiovascular diseases, including miscellaneous circulatory diseases, other heart diseases, hypertensive heart disease, and general arteriosclerosis.

Other Cancer Sites. Pipe smoking appears to be causally related to lip cancer. Cigarette smoking is a significant factor in the causation of cancer of the larynx. The evidence supports the belief that an association exists between tobacco use and cancer of the esophagus, and between cigarette smoking and cancer of the urinary bladder in men, but the data are not adequate to decide whether these relationships are causal. Data on an association between smoking and cancer of the stomach are contradictory and incomplete.

The Tobacco Habit and Nicotine

The habitual use of tobacco is related primarily to psychological and social drives, reinforced and perpetuated by the pharmacological actions of nicotine.

Social stimulation appears to play a major role in a young person's early and first experiments with smoking. No scientific evidence supports the popular hypothesis that smoking among adolescents is an expression of rebellion against authority. Individual stress appears to be associated more with fluctuations in the amount of smoking than with the prevalence of smoking. The overwhelming evidence indicates that smoking—its beginning, habituation, and occasional discontinuation—is to a very large extent psychologically and socially determined.

Nicotine is rapidly changed in the body to relatively inactive substances with low toxicity. The chronic toxicity of small doses of nicotine is low in experimental animals. These two facts, when taken in conjunction with the low mortality ratios of pipe and cigar smokers, indicate that the chronic toxicity of nicotine in quantities absorbed from smoking and other methods of tobacco use is very low and probably does not represent an important health hazard.

The significant beneficial effects of smoking occur primarily in the area of mental health, and the habit originates in a search for contentment. Since no means of measuring the quantity of these benefits is apparent, the Committee finds no basis for a judgment which would weigh benefits against hazards of smoking as it may apply to the general population.

On the basis of prolonged study and evaluation of many lines of converging evidence, the Committee makes the following judgment:

Cigarette smoking is a health hazard of sufficient importance in the United States to warrant appropriate remedial action.

U.S. Department of Health, Education, and Welfare, "Smoking and Health: Report of the Advisory Committee to the Surgeon General of the Public Health Service," 1964, http://www.cdc.gov/tobacco/sgr_1964/sgr64.htm.

Document 3: Selected Excerpts from Tobacco Industry Documents

In the 1990s, many thousands of secret tobacco industry documents were made public. Many of these documents cast the tobacco industry in a very poor light. Until that point, industry executives had claimed that nicotine was not addictive and that they did not intentionally market cigarettes to minors. The documents made it clear that as far back as the 1960s cigarette companies had known that nicotine was an addictive drug, and had knowingly profited from the popularity of certain cigarette brands among teenage smokers. This evidence of the industry's deception made it more vulnerable to lawsuits from both state governments and private individuals. A few of the most damning industry documents are quoted below.

Nicotine as a Drug

"Moreover, *nicotine* is addictive. We are, then, in the business of selling *nicotine*, an addictive drug in the release of stress mechanisms."

—July 1963 report from Brown and Williamson general counsel/vice president Addison Yeaman

"Do we really want to tout cigarette smoke as a drug? It is, of course."

—February 1969 memo from a Philip Morris researcher

"We have, then, as our first premise, that the primary motivation for smoking is to obtain the pharmacological effect of nicotine."

—1969 Philip Morris document entitled "Why One Smokes"

"Very few customers are aware of the effects of nicotine, i.e., its addictive nature and that nicotine is a poison."

—1978 Brown and Williamson document

"Let's face facts: Cigarette smoke is biologically active. Nicotine is a potent pharmacological agent. Every toxicologist, physiologist, medical doctor and most chemists know that. It's not a secret."

—1982 memo by Philip Morris researcher Thomas Osdene

Nicotine Manipulation

"We have a research program in process to obtain, by genetic means, any level of nicotine desired. . . . I think we can say even now that we can regulate, fairly precisely, the nicotine and sugar levels to almost any desired level management might require."

—1963 memo from a Brown and Williamson researcher

"The most direct solution to the problem of increasing nicotine delivery in the new product would be to add nicotine alkaloid directly to the tobaccos used in the new blend. The direct approach involves determining at which point in the manufacturing process the nicotine could be added, and secondly, determining where the necessary quantity of nicotine to support a major brand could be obtained. The direct approach involves some serious problems, mainly centering around the intensely poisonous nature of nicotine alkaloid."

—April 1977 report by Lorillard official H.J. Minnemeyer

"The view has been elaborated that nicotine is the primary reinforcer of continued smoking, and that this reinforcement value is in large part due to the functional contribution that the arousal modifying properties of nicotine makes to the negotiation of everyday life (coping). Two major research objectives are seen to be appropriate: 1) Fuller understanding of the effects of manipulating nicotine to tar ratio in cigarettes otherwise equated on all parameters. Such inquiry should be closely linked to the contribution of nicotine manipulations (i.e., enhanced nicotine to tar ratios) to producing cigarette designs which require less effort to deliver the required reward."

—September 1985 British-American Tobacco memo

Youth Smoking

"Marlboro's phenomenal growth rate in the past has been attributable in large part to our high market penetration among young smokers . . . 15 to 19 years old. . . . My own data, which includes younger teenagers, shows even higher Marlboro market penetration among 15–17-year-olds."

—May 1975 Philip Morris document

"Evidence is now available to indicate that the 14–18-year-old group is an increasing segment of the smoking population. RJR-T must soon establish a successful new brand in this market if our position in the industry is to be maintained in the long term."

—March 1976 R.J. Reynolds report

"The base of our business is the high school student."

—1978 Lorillard memo from executive T.L. Achey to former Lorillard president Curtis Judge

"The success of Marlboro Red during its most rapid growth period was because it became the brand of choice among teenagers who then stuck with it as they grew older."

—March 1981 Philip Morris report entitled "Young Smokers: Prevalence, Trends, Implications, and Related Demographic Trends"

"Because of our high share of the market among the youngest smokers, Philip Morris will suffer more than the other companies from the decline in the number of teenage smokers."

—March 1981 Philip Morris document

The tobacco industry documents are available from a variety of sources. Many of the Brown and Williamson documents are quoted in Stanton A. Glantz et al., *The Cigarette Papers.* Berkeley and Los Angeles: University of California Press, 1996. Over thirty-nine thousand documents subpoenaed in 1998 in the case of *State of Minnesota et al. v. Philip Morris, Inc.* are available on the U.S. House of Representatives Committee on Commerce website at http://www.house.gov/commerce/TobaccoDocs/documents.html. The website http://www.tobaccodocuments.org also provides a searchable index of documents.

Document 4: Selected Policies of the American Medical Association

Since the evidence on the health risks of smoking began to accumulate in the 1950s and 1960s, doctors have become active in efforts to reduce smoking and raise awareness of its dangers. The American Medical Association (AMA) has issued a variety of policy statements, clarifying its views on smoking and public health, several of which are reprinted below.

Tobacco as a Drug

It is the belief of the AMA that tobacco is a raw form of the drug nicotine and therefore is an addictive, crude drug. (Res. 408, A-93)

Environmental Tobacco Smoke (ETS)

Health Effects and Prevention Policies: The AMA: (1) supports classification of environmental tobacco smoke as a known human carcinogen; (2) urges that available evidence indicates that passive smoke exposure is associated with increased risk of sudden infant death syndrome and of cardiovascular disease; and (3) encourages physicians and medical societies to take a leadership role in defending the health of the public from ETS risks and from political assaults by the tobacco industry. (CSA Rep. 3, A-94; Reaffirmation A-99)

Tobacco Product Advertisements

The AMA (1) urges the 100 most widely circulating newspapers and the 100 most widely circulating magazines in the country that have not already done so to refuse to accept tobacco product advertisements, and (2) continues to support efforts by physicians and the public to persuade those media that accept tobacco product advertising to refuse such advertising. (Res. 76, I-80; Reaffirmed: CLRPD Rep. B, I-90)

Smoking and the Entertainment Industry

The AMA encourages the entertainment industry to continue to de-emphasize the role of smoking on television and in the movies. The AMA will aggressively lobby appropriate entertainment, sports, and fashion industry executives, the media and related trade associations to cease the use of tobacco products, trademarks and logos in their activities, productions, advertisements, and media accessible to minors. (Res. 24, I-86; Reaffirmed: Sunset Report, I-96; Appended Res. 426, I-97)

State Excise Taxes on Tobacco Products

The AMA will work for and encourage other interested groups to support efforts to pass increased excise taxes on tobacco products, with the proceeds used to support education and counter-advertising efforts. (Sub. Res. 555, A-92)

Regulation of Tobacco Products by the Food and Drug Administration
The AMA supports the regulation of tobacco products by the FDA. (Res. 243, A-89; Reaffirmed in lieu of Res. 232, I-94; Sub. Res. 406, I-95; Reaffirmation I-96)
American Medical Association website, http://www.ama-assn.org.

Document 5: The 2000 Surgeon General's Report on Reducing Tobacco Use

In 2000 Surgeon General David Satcher released a new report on smoking, entitled "Reducing Tobacco Use." The report evaluates the effectiveness of educational, clinical, regulatory, economic, and comprehensive approaches to tobacco use. The report's major findings are summarized in a Centers for Disease Control and Prevention fact sheet, which is excerpted below.

- Efforts to prevent the onset or continuance of tobacco use face the pervasive, countervailing influence of tobacco promotion by the tobacco industry, a promotion that takes place despite overwhelming evidence of adverse health effects from tobacco use.
- The available approaches to reducing tobacco use—educational, clinical, regulatory, economic, and comprehensive—differ substantially in their techniques and in the metric by which success can be measured. A hierarchy of effectiveness is difficult to construct.
- Approaches with the largest span of impact (economic, regulatory, and comprehensive) are likely to have the greatest long-term, population impact. Those with a smaller span of impact (educational and clinical) are of greater importance in helping individuals resist or abandon the use of tobacco.
- Each of the modalities reviewed provides evidence of effectiveness.
  - Educational strategies, conducted in conjunction with community- and media-based activities, can postpone or prevent smoking onset in 20 to 40 percent of adolescents.
  - Pharmacologic treatment of nicotine addiction, combined with behavioral support, will enable 20 to 25 percent of users to remain abstinent at one year posttreatment. Even less intense measures, such as physicians advising their patients to quit smoking, can produce cessation proportions of 5 to 10 percent.
  - Regulation of advertising and promotion, particularly that directed at young people, is very likely to reduce both prevalence and uptake of tobacco use.
  - Clean air regulations and restriction of minors' access to tobacco products contribute to a changing social norm with regard to smoking and may influence prevalence directly.

- An optimal level of excise taxation on tobacco products will reduce the prevalence of smoking, the consumption of tobacco, and the long-term health consequences of tobacco use.
- The impact of these various efforts, as measured with a variety of techniques, is likely to be underestimated because of the synergistic effect of these modalities. The potential for combined effects underscores the need for comprehensive approaches.
- State tobacco control programs, funded by excise taxes on tobacco products and settlements with the tobacco industry, have produced early, encouraging evidence of the efficacy of the comprehensive approach to reducing tobacco use.

Centers for Disease Control and Prevention, "Preventing Tobacco Use Among Young People: A Report of the Surgeon General: At-a-Glance," 1994, www.cdc.gov/tobacco/94oshaag.htm.

ORGANIZATIONS TO CONTACT

The editors have compiled the following list of organizations concerned with the issues debated in this book. The descriptions are derived from materials provided by the organizations. All have publications or information available for interested readers. The list was compiled on the date of publication of the present volume; the information provided here may change. Be aware that many organizations take several weeks or longer to respond to inquiries, so allow as much time as possible.

Action on Smoking and Health (ASH)
2013 H St. NW, Washington, DC 20006
(202) 659-4310
website: www.ash.org

ASH promotes the rights of nonsmokers and works to protect them from the harms of smoking. ASH worked to eliminate tobacco ads from radio and television and to ban smoking in public places. The organization publishes the bimonthly newsletter *ASH Smoking and Health Review* and its website posts news and fact sheets on a variety of topics, including teen smoking, passive smoking, and nicotine addiction.

American Cancer Society
1599 Clifton Road NE, Atlanta, GA 30329
(800) ACS-2345 (227-2345)
website: www.cancer.org

The American Cancer Society is one of the primary organizations in the United States devoted to educating the public about cancer and to funding cancer research. The society devotes a great deal of its resources to educating the public about the dangers of smoking and on lobbying for antismoking legislation. The society's website contains a section on tobacco control that includes reports, surveys, and position papers.

American Council on Science and Health (ACSH)
1995 Broadway, 2nd Floor, New York, NY 10023-5860
(212) 362-7044 • fax: (212) 362-4919
website: www.acsh.org

ACSH is a consumer education group concerned with issues related to food and nutrition, chemicals and pharmaceuticals, tobacco, the environment, and health. It opposes junk science that either ignores or exaggerates the evidence on the dangers of smoking. It publishes the quarterly magazine *Priorities* as well as the books *Cigarettes: What the Warning Label Doesn't Tell You* and *Environmental Tobacco Smoke: Health Risk or Health Hype?*

American Lung Association (ALA)
1740 Broadway, New York, NY 10019
(212) 315-8700
website:www.lungusa.org

ALA works to fight lung disease in all its forms, with special emphasis on asthma, tobacco control, and environmental health. ALA offers a variety of smoking control and prevention programs. It supports tobacco control initiatives, and its website offers information on state and federal tobacco control legislation.

Americans for Nonsmokers' Rights (ANR)
2530 San Pablo Ave., Suite J, Berkeley, CA 94702
(510) 841-3032 • fax: (510) 841-3060
website: www.no-smoke.org

ANR seeks to protect the rights of nonsmokers in the workplace and other public settings. It promotes smoking prevention, nonsmokers' rights, and public education about involuntary smoking. The organization publishes the quarterly newsletter *ANR Update*, the book *Clearing the Air*, and the guidebook *How to Butt In: Teens Take Action*.

American Smokers Alliance (ASA)
PO Box 189, Bellvue, CO 80512
website: www.smokers.org

ASA is a nonprofit organization of volunteers who believe that non-smokers and smokers have equal rights. ASA strives to unify existing smokers' rights efforts, combat anti-tobacco legislation, fight discrimination against smokers in the workplace, and encourage individuals to become involved in local smokers' rights movements. It maintains an archive on its website of articles that present smoking in an objective or positive light.

Campaign for Tobacco-Free Kids
1707 L St. NW, Suite 800, Washington, DC 20036
(202) 296-5469 • fax: (202) 296-5427
website: www.tobaccofreekids.org

The Campaign for Tobacco-Free Kids is the largest private initiative ever launched to protect children from tobacco addiction. The campaign works in partnership with government and nonprofit organizations to raise awareness about youth smoking and support tobacco control legislation. Among the center's numerous online publications are press releases, fact sheets, and reports, including *Big Tobacco: Still Addicting Kids*, and *Behind the Smokescreen*.

Canadian Council for Tobacco Control (CCTC)
170 Laurier Ave. W, Suite 1000, Ottawa, ON K1P 5V5 CANADA
(800) 267-5234 • (613) 567-3050 • fax: (613) 567-5695
website: www.cctc.ca/ncth

The CCTC works to ensure a healthier society, free from addiction and involuntary exposure to tobacco products. It promotes a comprehensive tobacco control program involving educational, social, fiscal, and legislative interventions. It publishes several fact sheets, including *Tobacco in Canada: A Statistical Overview* and *Promoting a Lethal Product*.

Centers for Disease Control and Prevention (CDC)
(800) 311-3435
Tobacco Information and Prevention Source (TIPS) website: www.cdc.gov/tobacco

The CDC is an agency of the federal Department of Health and Human Services. The CDC's Office on Smoking and Health, in conjunction with the Office of the Surgeon General, works to reduce smoking in order to help people lead long and healthy lives. CDC's TIPS website contains online versions of all surgeons general reports on smoking, as well as fact sheets, graphs, and special reports on smoking.

Children Opposed to Smoking Tobacco (COST)
Mary Volz School, 509 W 3rd Ave., Runnemede, NJ 08078
e-mail: costkids@costkids.org • website: www.costkids.org

COST was founded in 1996 by a group of middle school students committed to keeping tobacco products out of the hands of children. Much of the organization's efforts are spent fighting the tobacco industry's advertising campaigns directed at children and teenagers. Articles such as "Environmental Tobacco Smoke," "What Is a Parent To Do?," and "What You Can Do" are available on its website.

Competitive Enterprise Institute (CEI)
1001 Connecticut Ave. NW, Suite 1250, Washington DC 20036
(202) 331-1010 • fax: (202) 331-0640
website: www.cei.org

The institute is a pro–free market public interest group involved in a wide range of issues, including tobacco. CEI questions the validity and accuracy of Environmental Protection Agency reports on secondhand smoke and opposes lawsuits against the tobacco industry. Its publications include books, monographs, and policy studies, and the monthly newsletter *CEI Update*.

drkoop.com
700 North Mopac, Suite 400, Austin, TX 78731
(512) 583-KOOP • fax: (512) 583-5727
e-mail: feedback@drkoop.com • website: www.drkoop.com/wellness/ tobacco

Based on the vision of former U.S. surgeon general C. Everett Koop, drkoop.com is a consumer-focused interactive website that provides users with comprehensive health-care information on a wide variety of subjects, including tobacco. The organization publishes reports, fact sheets, press releases, and books, including *The No-Nag, No-Guilt, Do-It-Your-Own-Way Guide to Quitting Smoking*.

Environmental Protection Agency (EPA)
Indoor Air Quality Information Clearinghouse
PO Box 37133, Washington, DC 20013-7133
(800) 438-4318 • (202) 484-1307 • fax: (202) 484-1510
e-mail: iaqinfo@aol.com • website: www.epa.gov/iaq

The EPA is the agency of the U.S. government that coordinates actions designed to protect the environment. It promotes indoor air quality standards that reduce the dangers of secondhand smoke. The EPA publishes and distributes reports such as *Setting the Record Straight: Secondhand Smoke Is a Preventable Health Risk, Respiratory Health Effects of Passive Smoking,* and *Children and Secondhand Smoke.*

Fight Ordinances & Restrictions to Control & Eliminate Smoking (FORCES)
PO Box 14347, San Francisco, CA 94114-0347
(415) 675-0157
website: www.forces.org

FORCES fights smoking ordinances and restrictions designed to eventually eliminate smoking, and works to increase public awareness of smoking-related legislation. It opposes state or local ordinances it deems unfair to those who choose to smoke. Although FORCES does not advocate smoking, it asserts that an individual has the right to choose to smoke and that smokers should be accommodated where and when possible. FORCES publishes *Tobacco Weekly* as well as many articles.

U.S. Food and Drug Administration (FDA)
Rockville, MD 20857
(800) 532-4440 • (301) 443-1130 • fax: (301) 443-9767
website: www.fda.gov

As the agency of the U.S. government charged with protecting the health of the public against impure and unsafe foods, drugs, cosmetics, and other potential hazards, the FDA has sought the regulation of nicotine as a drug and has investigated manipulation of nicotine levels in cigarettes by the tobacco industry. It provides copies of congressional testimony given in the debate over the regulation of nicotine.

FOR FURTHER READING

Stanton A. Glantz et al., *The Cigarette Papers*. Berkeley and Los Angeles: University of California Press, 1996. A compendium and interpretation of the documents taken from the cigarette company Brown and Williamson by whistle-blower Merrell Williams.

Eileen Heyes, *Tobacco U.S.A.: The Industry Behind the Smoke Curtain.* Brookfield, CT: Millbrook Press, 1999. A concise overview of tobacco use in America, with an emphasis on how the tobacco industry has continued to deny the health risks of smoking.

Richard Kluger, *Ashes to Ashes: America's Hundred-Year Cigarette War, the Public Health, and the Unabashed Triumph of Philip Morris.* New York : Vintage Books, 1997. This sweeping history of smoking in America gives special attention to the role of the largest U.S. tobacco company.

Edward L. Koven, *Smoking: The Story Behind the Maze*. Commack, NY: Kroshka Books, 1998. The author attacks the tobacco industry as deceitful and even criminal and offers proposals for reducing smoking, including higher taxes on cigarettes, bans on tobacco advertising, and restrictions on smoking in public places.

Rachel Kranz, *Straight Talk About Smoking*. New York: Facts On File, 1999. This book is intended to provide young adults with clear, unbiased information with which to make decisions about smoking.

Susan S. Lang and Beth H. Marks, *Teens and Tobacco: A Fatal Attraction*. New York: Twenty-First Century Books, 1996. This fact-filled book aimed at teens emphasizes the dangers of youth smoking and the methods by which advertising targets teens.

Mike Males, *Smoked: Why Joe Camel Is Still Smiling*. Monroe, ME: Common Courage Press, 1999. The author contends that efforts to restrict the marketing of cigarettes to teens in the 1990s have been ineffective and sometimes counterproductive.

Jeffrey A. Schaler and Magda E. Schaler, eds., *Smoking: Who Has the Right?* Amherst, NY: Prometheus Books, 1998. The essays in this anthology focus on government regulation of smoking; many of them argue against tobacco control measures.

Jacob Sullum, *The Antismoking Crusade and the Tyranny of Public Health*. New York: Simon & Schuster, 1998. An attack on the science of secondhand smoke and a case against regulating smoking in the name of public health.

Works Consulted

Books

Laura K. Egendorf, ed., *Teens at Risk: Opposing Viewpoints.* San Diego: Greenhaven Press, 1997.

James D. Torr, ed., *Alcoholism: Current Controversies.* San Diego: Greenhaven Press, 2000.

———, *Health Care: Opposing Viewpoints.* San Diego: Greenhaven Press, 2000.

Carol Wekesser, ed., *Smoking: Current Controversies.* San Diego: Greenhaven Press, 1997.

Mary E. Williams, ed., *Smoking: At Issue.* San Diego: Greenhaven Press, 2000.

Mary E. Williams and Tamara L. Roleff, eds., *Tobacco and Smoking: Opposing Viewpoints.* San Diego: Greenhaven Press, 1998.

Periodicals

Fred Barbash, "Warning: Zealotry May Be Hazardous to Your Health," *Washington Post*, April 27, 1998.

Jan J. Barendregt, Luc Bonneux, and Paul J. van der Maas, "The Health Care Costs of Smoking," *New England Journal of Medicine*, October 9, 1997.

Joan Biskupic, "Legislation by Litigation," *Washington Post*, September 3, 1999.

John E. Calfee, "Why the War on Tobacco Will Fail," *Weekly Standard*, July 20, 1998.

CQ Researcher, "Closing in on Tobacco," November 12, 1999.

Ronald M. Davis, "Exposure to Environmental Tobacco Smoke: Identifying and Protecting Those at Risk," *JAMA*, December 9, 1998.

Economist, "When Lawsuits Make Policy," November 21, 1998.

Ellen Goodman, "Whining Tobacco Companies Still Targeting Youth," *Liberal Opinion Week*, April 20, 1998.

Gayle M.B. Hanson, "Tobacco and Liberty," *Insight on the News*, March 16, 1998.

John Fraser Hart and Ennis L. Chang, "Turmoil in Tobaccoland," *Geographical Review*, October 1996.

Thomas Houston and Nancy J. Kaufman, "Tobacco Control in the 21st Century," *JAMA*, August 9, 2000.

Issues and Controversies on File, "Tobacco Litigation," March 7, 1997.

David A. Kessler, "Time to Act on Cigarettes," *Washington Post*, April 10, 2000.

C. Everett Koop, David A. Kessler, and George D. Lundberg, "Reinventing American Tobacco Policy," *JAMA*, February 18, 1998.

Quoted in Marianne Lavelle, "Teen Tobacco Wars," *U.S. News & World Report*, February 7, 2000.

Robert A. Levy, "The Tobacco Deal: Myths and Misconceptions," *Freeman*, January 1998.

————, "When Theft Masquerades as Law," *Cato Policy Report*, March/April 2000.

Robert A. Levy and Rosalind B. Marimont, "Lies, Damned Lies, and 400,000 Smoking-Related Deaths," *Regulation*, April 1999.

John J. Lynch, "Do We Need a Tobacco Bill? Emphatically Yes, and Now," *World & I*, July 1998.

Anne Platt McGinn, "The Nicotine Cartel," *Worldwatch*, July/August 1997.

Minneapolis Star-Tribune, "Study Links Marketing, Teen Smoking," October 18, 1995.

————, "Tobacco Goes on Trial," January 18, 1998.

Mother Jones, "The Tobacco Wars," May/June 1996.

National Review, "Public Policy: Legal Muggings," April 17, 2000.

Jay Nordlinger, "Secondhand Statistics," *Weekly Standard*, August 3, 1998.

Bill Novelli, "Should the FDA Assume Regulatory Power over Tobacco Products? Yes: An Agency Free from Political Influence Is Situated to Rein in this Rogue Industry," *Insight on the News*, May 10, 1999.

John Parascandola, "The Surgeon General and Smoking," *Public Health Reports*, September/October 1997.

Dennis Prager, "The Soul-Corrupting Anti-Tobacco Crusade," *Weekly Standard*, July 20, 1998.

Robert J. Samuelson, "The Amazing Smoke Screen," *Newsweek*, November 30, 1998.

Jacob Sullum, "Smoke Alarm," *Reason*, May 1996.

———, "Whose Risk Is It, Anyway?" *New York Times*, February 19, 1999.

David Tannenbaum, "Smoking Guns I: Marketing to Kids," *Multinational Monitor*, July/August 1998.

———, "Smoking Guns II: Nicotine Manipulation," *Multinational Monitor*, July/August 1998.

James Taranto, "An Adolescent View of Smoking," *American Enterprise*, September/October 1998.

Stuart Taylor Jr., "Tobacco Lawsuits: Taxing the Victims to Enrich the Lawyers," *National Journal*, July 29, 2000.

Quoted in Ira Teinowitz, "Just Take the Money and Run (the Ads)," *Washington Post*, December 14, 1998.

David Tell, "A New Direction on the Tobacco Road," *Weekly Standard*, May 5, 1997.

Internet Resources

Advisory Committee on Tobacco Policy and Public Health, "Summary of the Major Recommendations of the Task Force on Environmental Tobacco Smoke," 1997, www.lungusa.org/tobacco/smkkoop.html.

American Cancer Society, "Cigarette Smoking and Cancer," March 30, 2000, www.cancer.org/tobacco.cigarette_smoking.html.

American Medical Association, *How to Help Patients Stop Smoking: Guidelines for Diagnosis and Treatment of Nicotine Dependence.* Chicago: American Medical Association, 1994, http://iumeded.med.iupui.edu/Tobacco/tobuse.htm.

Joseph A. Califano Jr., opening address at Substance Abuse in the 21st Century: Positioning the Nation for Progress, Simi Valley, California, March 1, 2000, www.casacolumbia.org.

Campaign for Tobacco-Free Kids, "The Cigarette Companies Cannot Survive Unless Kids Smoke," July 18, 2000, http://tobaccofreekids.org/research/factsheets/pdf/0012.pdf.

———, "In the Tobacco Industry's Own Words: Nicotine as a Drug," http://tobaccofreekids.org/research/factsheets/pdf/0009.pdf.

Centers for Disease Control and Prevention, "History of the 1964 Surgeon General's Report on Smoking and Health," July 1996, www.cdc.gov/tobacco/31yrsgen.htm.

———, "In the 30 Years Since the First Surgeon General's Report . . ." www.cdc.gov/tobacco/30yrs2t.htm.

———, "Preventing Tobacco Use Among Young People: A Report of the Surgeon General: At-a-Glance," 1994, www.cdc.gov/tobacco/94oshaag.htm.

———, "Reducing Tobacco Use: A Report of the Surgeon General: At-a-Glance," 2000, www.cdc.gov/tobacco/sgr_tobacco_pdf/aag2cpy.pdf.

———, "Tobacco Information and Prevention Source: Overview," www.cdc.gov/tobacco/issue.htm.

Environmental Protection Agency, "Setting the Record Straight: Secondhand Smoke Is a Preventable Health Risk," June 1994, www.epa.gov/iaq/pubs/strsfs.html.

Wanda Hamilton, "What Shall We Do About the Kids?: A Selected Bibliography on Underage Tobacco Use," National Smokers Alliance, 1999, www.smokersalliance.org/hamilton1.html.

Judith Hatton, "Smoking and Addiction," *Free Choice*, January/February 1996, http://forest-on-smoking.org.uk/factsheets/aaddict.htm.

Mark Lender, "Born Again: The Resurgence of American Prohibition," *Ideas on Liberty*, March 1996, www.fee.org/freeman/96/9604/lender.html.

Robert A. Levy and Rosalind B. Marimont, "Blowing Smoke About Tobacco-Related Deaths," *Cato Today's Commentary*, April 29, 1999, www.cato.org/dailys/04-29-99.html.

Rosalind B. Marimont, "War on Smoking," 1997. Brochure distributed by FORCES USA, www.forces.org/articles/files/roz-03.htm.

National Cancer Institute, "Environmental Tobacco Smoke," February 14, 2000, http://cancernet.nci.nih.gov/cancer_types/lung_cancer.shtml.

National Institute on Drug Abuse, "Nicotine Addiction," July 24, 1998, www.nida.nih.gov/researchreports/nicotine/nicotine.html.

Robert Peck, "Is Cigarette Advertising Protected by the First Amendment? Yes," *Priorities*, vol. 5, no.3, 1993, www.acsh.org/publications.priorities/0503/pcpyes.html.

Martha Perkse, "Does Smoking Really Cause over 400,000 Deaths per Year in the U.S.?" www.forces.org/evidence/files/martha2.html.

David Satcher, "The Surgeon General's Report on Reducing Tobacco Use: Tobacco Advertising and Promotion Fact Sheet," 2000, www.cdc.gov/tobacco/sgr_tobacco_pdf/TobaccoAdvertising.pdf.

Jon Saunders, "The Tyranny of the Proper," *Ideas on Liberty*, December 1998, www.fee.org/freeman/98/9812/happiness.html.

Jacob Sullum, "Blowing Smoke About Addiction, Ability to Quit," *Reason*, May 25, 1997, www.reason.com/opeds/jacob052597.html.

————, "Cowboys, Camels, and Kids: Does Advertising Turn People into Smokers?" *Reason*, April 1998, www.reason.com/9804/fe.sullum.html.

Elizabeth M. Whelan, "Warning: Overstating the Case Against Secondhand Smoke Is Unnecessary—and Harmful to Public Health Policy," American Council on Science and Health editorial, August 1, 2000, www.acsh.org/press/editorials/warning080100.html.

Larry C. White, "Is Cigarette Advertising Protected by the First Amendment? No," *Priorities*, vol. 5, no. 3, 1993, www.acsh.org/publications/priorities/0503/pcpno.html.

INDEX

advertising
claims of, 49
cost of, 45
denial of link to cancers and, 10–11
encourages smoking, 45–46
con, 52–53
in Europe, 73, 80
impacts brand preferences only,
45–46, 53–54
against McCain bill, 15
regulation of, 12, 15, 47, 63
helps Big Tobacco, 80
is constitutional
con, 81
should be banned, 73–74
effects of, 50
targets teenagers, 34–35, 46–49
con, 53–54
for unhealthful products, 68
alcohol use, 9, 34, 82
American Civil Liberties Union, 81
American Law Institute, 52
American Lung Association (ALA),
12
American Medical Association, 10
antismoking campaigns
are effective, 76
con, 42
are not governmental functions, 40
described, 40, 75–76
should target teenagers, 36
con, 40–41
Armentano, D.T., 53

Bailey, William Everett, 45
Barbash, Fred, 68
Big Tobacco
crusade against is political, 30, 31
encourages smoking, 45
lied to public about
addictive powers of nicotine, 60
link between lung cancer and
smoking, 58–59
public opinion about, 58
see also lawsuits
Biskupic, Joan, 56
Brown and Williamson, 46–47, 58

Calfee, John E., 53
Califano, Joseph A., 33
California
antismoking campaigns in, 40, 76
ban on smoking in bars in, 13, 28,
75
Environmental Protection Agency,
74
lawsuit ban in, 52
teenage smoking in, 42
Camel, 48, 49
Campaign for Tobacco-Free Kids,
35, 39, 46, 61, 76
Canada, 73
cancers
are caused by smoking, 19, 20
annual deaths, 21
con, 27
lung
Big Tobacco knowledge of link to
smoking, 58–59
increase in, 10
is very rare among smokers, 30
secondhand smoke and, 11, 23,
79
cardiovascular diseases
are caused by smoking, 19
annual deaths, 21
con, 27, 68
secondhand smoke and, 23
*Case Against the Little White Slaver,
The* (Ford), 9
Centers for Disease Control and
Prevention (CDC), 11, 20–21,
26–27, 32, 41–42, 49
Chafetz, Morris E., 54
Chang, Ennis L., 8
Chapman, Stephen, 64
Charen, Mona, 54–55
cigarettes
filtered, 10
flavored, 48
Cipollone v. Liggett Group, 13
Clean Indoor Air Act, 12
Clinton, Bill, 15, 61, 68
Council for Tobacco Research
(CTR), 58–59

Davis, Ronald M., 74
deaths
  annual, 21
  are wrongly attributed to smoking,
    26–27
  decrease cost of health care, 65
  due to secondhand smoke, 74
  rate of, 19–20
Denmark, 73
drugs, illegal, 34, 40–41
Duke, James B., 8

Economist (magazine), 68
Edison, Thomas, 9
Elders, Joycelyn, 50
Environmental Protection Agency
  (EPA), 23, 28, 29
environmental tobacco smoke
  (ETS). *See* secondhand smoke
Europe, 73, 80
Eysenck, Hans, 54

Florida, 51
Food and Drug Administration
  (FDA), 36, 71–72
Foote, Emerson, 46
Ford, Henry, 9
For Your Own Good: The Anti-
  Smoking Crusade and the Tyranny of
  Public Health (Sullum), 81
"Frank Statement to Smokers, A,"
  10–11

Goodman, Ellen, 36

Hamilton, Wanda, 42–43
Hanson, Gayle M.B., 67
Hart, John Fraser, 8
health
  costs of care, 61
    are inflated, 65
    smoking saves government
      money, 65
  risks are serious, 11, 19, 33
    con, 26
      lowers risk of Parkinson's
        disease, 30–31
  see also secondhand smoke; *specific*
    diseases
Health and Human Services,
  Department of, 32, 38

heart disease. *See* cardiovascular
  diseases
Henley, Patricia, 51, 55
Henningfield, Jack, 22
Houston, Thomas, 73

India, 73
"Industry Response to the Cigarette
  Health Controversy" (Pepples), 59
Insight on the News (magazine), 67
Internet, 47–48
Invisible Drug, The (Bailey), 45

Joe Camel, 15, 47, 49
Journal of Marketing, 49
Journal of the American Medical
  Association (JAMA), 39, 57

Kaufman, Nancy J., 73
Kessler, David A., 22, 57, 61, 72
Kool, 47
Koop, C. Everett, 19, 57, 61
Koven, Edward L., 57–58

Lang, Susan S., 34–35, 36, 49
lawsuits
  are justified, 56
    con, 63
  attorneys' fees from, 64
  class-action, 51–52, 57–58
  federal, 15
  history of, 56–57
  right to sue and, 13
  set a dangerous precedent, 67–68
  state, 14, 51, 58
    settlements, 56
      do not benefit public, 67
      have effect of legislation, 63
      have not hurt Big Tobacco,
        65–67
      restrict advertising, 15, 47
Lender, Mark, 82
Leshner, Alan I., 22
Levy, Robert A., 27, 31, 41, 64, 67,
  82
Lorillard Tobacco, 47
Los Angeles Times (newspaper), 42
Lundberg, George D., 57, 61
Lynch, John J., 73, 76

Marimont, Rosalind B., 27, 29, 31, 41

Marks, Beth H., 34–35, 36, 49
Marlboro, 46
Marlboro Man, 48, 49
Massachusetts, 51, 76
McCain, John, 14
McGinn, Anne Platt, 32, 33
Medicare, 15, 61
Merchants of Death: The American Tobacco Industry (White), 74
Minnesota
  ban on smoking in public places in, 12
  lawsuit by, 14, 51, 58
Mississippi, 14, 51
Monitoring the Future, 32, 38
Murray, David, 29
Myers, Matthew, 48–49

National Cancer Institute, 23
National Institute on Drug Abuse, 21
National Journal, 66
National Review (magazine), 63
National Tobacco Policy and Youth Smoking Reduction Act (McCain bill), 14–15
Native Americans, 8
New England Journal of Medicine, 65
Newport, 49
Newsweek (magazine), 80
nicotine
  concentrations in cigarettes, 60
  FDA should regulate, 36, 71–72
  is addictive, 11, 13, 34
    Big Tobacco knowledge of, 60
    claim benefits many industries, 30
    claim harms war against illegal drugs, 40–41
    con, 29–30, 54–55
    mechanism described, 21–22
  levels of, 10
  regulation of, 71–72
Nordlinger, Jay, 39
Novelli, Bill, 72

Osteen, William J., 29

Peck, Robert, 81
Pepples, Ernest, 59
Philip Morris, 46, 47, 51, 52, 58
Pierce, John, 49
Prager, Dennis, 40–41, 54

Preventive Medicine (journal), 72–73
Pro-Children Act, 12
Prohibition, 9, 82

RAND Corporation, 30
Reason (magazine), 9, 30, 52
"Reducing Tobacco Use" (Surgeon General's Report of 2000), 79–80
reproductive health of women, 20
respiratory diseases
  are caused by smoking, 19, 20
  annual deaths, 21
  secondhand smoke and, 23
R.J. Reynolds, 48
Rolling Stone (magazine), 48
Roosevelt, Franklin D., 10

Samuelson, Robert J., 80
Satcher, David, 45
Saunders, Jon, 78
Schaler, Jeffrey A., 55, 68, 81
Schuh, Leslie M., 22
secondhand smoke
  deaths due to, 74
  described, 23
  is hazardous to health, 23
    con, 29, 79
  lung cancer and, 11, 79
Smith, Guy, 46
smoking
  begins in teen years, 33, 46
  history of, 8–10, 52
  is habit, 29–30
  is issue of individual choice, 51, 68, 78, 81–82
  quitting
    increased taxes promote, 73
    proves that nicotine is not addictive, 29, 54–55
    rate of, 21
  rate of, 11, 32
    by adults, 20–21
    antismoking campaigns and, 42, 76
    by teenagers, 32, 38, 42–43
    is exaggerated, 39–40
  reasons for, 46, 53, 54
  regulation of
    advertisements. *See* advertising
    federal
      in day-care centers and schools, 12

failure of McCain bill, 15
legislation
    is proper approach, 64
    should be enforced, 35–36, 79
    state, 12, 13, 28, 75
    warning labels, 11–12
should be banned in public places,
    74–75
Smoking: The Story Behind the Maze
    (Koven), 57
*State of Minnesota et al. v. Philip
    Morris, Inc.*, 58
Stevens, Colleen, 75
stroke. *See* cardiovascular diseases
Sullum, Jacob, 9, 30, 52, 53, 81
Supreme Court
    ban on cigarettes and, 9
    Cipollone v. Liggett Group, 13
    regulation of advertising and,
        73–74
    regulation of nicotine and, 36, 72
surgeon general's reports
    of 1964, 11, 19, 30–31
    of 1986, 11
    of 1988, 11, 21
    of 1994, 33, 34
    of 2000, 50, 79–80

Taranto, James, 41
taxes
    amount of, 64
    are form of social control, 80
    hurt the poor, 80
    internationally, 73
    reduce smoking, 35
    should be increased, 35, 72–73
    to fund antismoking campaigns,
        75–76
Taylor, Stuart, Jr., 66
teenagers
    advertising targets, 34–35, 46–49
    con, 53–54
    antismoking campaigns should
        target, 36

con, 40–41
brands smoked by, 46–47, 49
smoking by
    illegal substance use and, 34
    is serious problem, 32
    con, 38, 41
    measures to reduce
        antismoking campaigns, 40
        enforce existing legislation,
            35–36, 79
        taxes, 35
    rate of, 32, 38, 42–43
        is exaggerated, 39–40
    reasons for, 34, 49
Teens and Tobacco: A Fatal Attraction
    (Lang and Marks), 34–35, 49
Tell, David, 64
Terry, Luther, 11, 19
tobacco
    economic importance of, 8, 10, 11
    see also Big Tobacco
    is harmful when used as intended, 76
Tobacco Industry Research
    Committee, 58
Tobacco Wars. *See* lawsuits
"Trends in Cigarette Smoking in the
    United States" (*JAMA*), 39
*Tyranny of Experts, The: Blowing the
    Whistle on the Cult of Experts*
    (Chafetz), 54

United Kingdom, 73

Washington Post (newspaper), 58, 68
Weekly Standard (newspaper), 39, 64
West Virginia, 51
Whelan, Elizabeth M., 23, 28, 79
White, Larry C., 74
Williams, Merrell, 13, 58
World Health Organization (WHO),
    29, 30, 79
World War II, 10

Yeaman, Addison, 60

ABOUT THE AUTHOR

James Torr has edited several Greenhaven books, including *Current Controversies: Medical Ethics* and *America's Decades: The 1980s*. He has also written *Euthanasia*, a title in the Opposing Viewpoints Digests series. He is currently working as a freelance writer and editor in Providence, Rhode Island.